THE DOLCE DIET

3 WEEKS TO SHREDDED

By MIKE DOLCE
with Brandy Roon

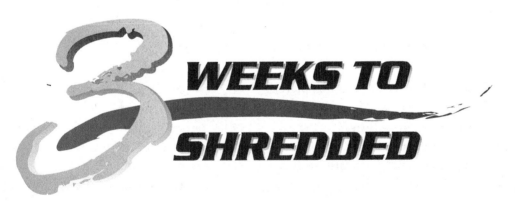

Conrad James Books
Las Vegas, NV
www.conradjamesbooks.com

 Published by Conrad James Books. First Edition. Printed in the United States of America.

ISBN 978-0-9849631-8-8

Edited by Brandy Roon & Sarah Veit
Cover Design: Zack Sherman
Cover Photo: Tom Bear
Interior Photos: Brandi Farra, Silton Buendia, Mike Dolce, Al Powers
Interior Layout & Illustrations: Brady Scott
Professional consultant: Samantha Wilkinson, MS, RDN, LD

TABLE OF CONTENTS

Part IV

Appendix

NOTE

You should seek medical supervision before beginning any diet or exercise program. Nothing written in this book should be taken as a substitute for medical advice. This book is for information purposes only. The publisher, author and all those involved with this book have done so with honest effort and make no representations with respect to the accuracy of its contents. None involved with the production and distribution of this book shall be held liable nor accountable for any loss or damage including but not limited to special, incidental, consequential or other. Mention of specific organizations, entities, individuals, companies or authorities does not imply endorsement by the author, publisher or any party involved with this book nor does mention of specific organizations, entities, individuals, companies or authorities imply that they endorse this book, its author, the publisher or any party involved with this book. Information within this book is general and offered with no guarantees on the part of the author, publisher or any party involved with this book.

INTRODUCTION

The question I'm most often asked besides, "What can I eat in place of vegetables?" is "Are you sure about this?!"

That question is asked by most every athlete the first time I work with them. I understand. They're nervous. They've had bad experiences cutting weight before. And the common belief is that they must suffer and starve themselves to make weight.

A failed weight cut can finish an athlete faster than a Ronda Rousey arm bar. It's a lot of pressure.

I know why they ask if I'm sure. Because they want to be sure. Because if I'm confident, they also can be confident. (And I'm always confident.) They want this process to be as simple as they've heard it is from their fellow athletes, from management, from the thousands of folks around the world who've used the Mike Dolce method to cut weight. What is that method exactly? You're about to find out.

In the first edition of 3 Weeks to Shredded I detailed exactly what I ate during the final 3 weeks of a 6-week fight camp in which I cut a total of 42.8 lbs. During the last 3 weeks, I cut 27.8 lbs. 3 Weeks to Shredded details those final 21 days. Let me be clear: Weight cuts, in general, are not healthy. That 2007 weight cut was extreme.

I have spent my 25-year career trying to perfect the weight-cutting process while maintaining optimal health.

Though I knew what I was doing then, just as I know what I'm doing now, my methods, like the evolution of man, change. The principles, however, stay the same.

The inspiration for the first edition of 3 Weeks to Shredded came during that monster cut in 2007. This may surprise you, but I wasn't inspired to write it down by the elite athletes I worked with. Instead, the constant questions from the ladies in my Women's FIT Class drove me to reveal the process. That's right. It was the soccer moms, CEOs, hair stylists and lawyers who came to my class 3 nights a week.

I walked in one day and the ladies took one look at me and shrieked. They'd seen me at the beginning of that fight camp at 212.8 lbs. Here I was just 5 weeks later weighing 180. I had lost 32 lbs. in those 5 weeks and would lose another 10 over the next 6 days.

"What happened to you?"

"What did you do?"

"How did you lose so much weight since last week?"

"Yeah, how did you lose weight?"

"What did you eat?"

"How did you train?"

During the next few classes, the questions kept coming. My wife, Brandy, finally said, "Let's just write down what you did and give it to whomever wants it." So we did.

I wrote down the process, detailing the meal plan that aided me during the last 3 weeks of that 42-lb. weight cut, along with the basic principles of goal setting and discipline I employed.

We made copies and handed them out at the next class. The requests for the manual kept coming and we kept handing it out, which got costly. So we ended up selling them. And sell they did! The process worked like no other anyone had ever come across.

Over the next few years, tens of thousands of orders came in from around the world and people reported back to us their amazing results. Instead of using the information in 3 Weeks to Shredded for a temporary weight cut, which was and still is the book's intended purpose, regular folks were "cutting weight" for weddings, high school reunions or just to jumpstart their bodies into an eventual transition of longterm healthy lifestyles.

Learning this, we decided to publish LIVING LEAN as a longterm lifestyle guide, emphasizing weight loss, muscle gain and overall health, while 3 Weeks to Shredded would remain solely a manual for weight cuts. Since the publication of the first edition of 3 Weeks to Shredded in 2007, I have continued my work with the world's most elite athletes, helping them lose weight, get in shape and compete at levels never before seen in sport. My methods have taken the pain out of the weight cut.

In this revised and expanded edition, I offer new tips and techniques to help you further your goal of getting in the absolute leanest possible condition, while focusing on your health and happiness.

Yes, you can be healthy, happy and SHREDDED!

This process is not for everyone, but 3 Weeks to Shredded works for every person who doesn't make excuses for why they can't do it. My personal results are certainly not typical.

In Part 1, you will learn the Dolce Diet Principles, a longevity-based approach to immediate weight loss and optimal performance. We teach you the importance of setting goals, the difference between a weight cut and weight loss, and how to maximize your success outside the gym.

In Part 2, you will learn about that 2007 weight cut, and in Part 3 I'll show you how that process has changed today based upon my continued experience working with world-class athletes.

In Part 4, we'll talk about the dangers of cutting weight, and troubleshoot challenges that may come up while traveling, or as a result of uninformed people around you who still insist on utilizing the outdated archaic methods commonly used to this day.

Equally as important to how we cut weight is how we put it back on. Here, we'll also talk about how to properly rehydrate, what to drink, what to eat and what to avoid at all costs.

3 Weeks to Shredded covers many of the principles that form the major foundation of my life's work, which is based on attaining vibrant health and exceeding physical limitations through nutrition and lifestyle management. I've experimented with weight gain and weight reduction over the past 25 years using myself and the greatest athletes in the world as proving grounds. Through trial and error, I've discovered what works and what doesn't. I suffered, so you won't have to. NOW LET'S GET SHREDDED!

PRAISE FOR THE DOLCE DIET: 3 WEEKS TO SHREDDED

Thanks to Mike Dolce I am sitting here today at a healthy 172 lbs. after weighing in last February 1 at 340 lbs. This is a new life that I've grown into with the help of Mike and The Dolce Diet. I strongly recommend the 3 Weeks to Shredded program. *-Justin Boyarski*

Completed 3 Weeks to Shredded this week and lost 38 lbs. Can't describe the feeling of being alive again. The difference you guys are making cannot be measured. *-Niall Hogan*

@TheDolceDiet works. I'm 100 lbs lighter & working out at an MMA gym. *-Christine Ashton @blu_vision*

I used your 3 Weeks to Shredded book and am having crazy results! You and Brandy are amazing people and the work you do has inspired me to major in exercise science and nutrition. Thank you for keeping a lot on my plate! I was 188 lbs. and 10% bodyfat. Two months later I'm 166.4 lbs. around 5.7% bodyfat and not planning on losing another percent! *-Michael Heckert*

I used 3 Weeks to Shredded and cut down from 163 lbs. to 145 lbs. with ease, and for the first time I did not use a sauna! At the weigh-ins, I knew I had already defeated my opponent. *-Dan Ige*

#HardWorkPaysOff 17 lbs. down in four weeks! Haven't felt this good since college soccer! Shout to The Dolce Diet - lifestyle change made easy *-Kathryn Wallis @wallis1181*

Since I've been following your principles I have not only put on muscle mass super fast, which is my goal, but have gained so much confidence and knowledge. I am a much happier and stress free person. I see everything in a completely different perspective. I ALSO have not had a single cold or any sort of sickness at all in a year now! Thanks to your guidance and motivation I have finally got the confidence to start training for my first fitness competition. *-Jordan Dobie*

Hi, I have started 3 Weeks to Shredded. I'm eating exactly what is on the list. I'm five days in and feel fantastic. I started at 115.7 kg. (255 lbs.) and I'm currently 112.0 kg (246 lbs.) this morning. *-T-Rex*

I have purchased 3 Weeks to Shredded and Living Lean. I started seven weeks ago and have went from 227 lbs. to 192 lbs. Your principles and guidelines are awesome. Real food all day long. *-Dwayne Mallon*

I started 3 Weeks to Shredded in January and then moved on to the cookbook. I love The Dolce Diet Principles. Since I started I have lost 20 lbs. and toned up with the help of UFC FIT. *-Susana Melissa Ramirez*

Just got 3 Weeks to Shredded. Gotta say I'm full of energy and it's day 4. *-Karl Mifsud*

So I had a bet with a friend starting in October that we would both get to 200 lbs. I was 220 and he was 225. FYI: I'm 5'9". Being lazy, I didn't do anything to change. I ordered your book the week before Thanksgiving. I gorged myself at Thanksgiving, weighing more than 220 lbs. I started your diet the next week. This Friday was Dec. 31 and weigh-in day. Earlier in the week I was waking up at 203 lbs. That morning I woke up at 203 and cut some water weight and BOOM - 195 lbs! The water weight came off so fast! I lost 2 inches around my waste - jeans falling off - I can fit into a 36 for the first time in YEARS! *-Danyo K.*

Down 16 lbs. in 8 days! @TheDolceDiet, thank you! I'm living lean, eating clean, and feeling mean! #teamdolce *-Ryan Gillett*

My journey with The Dolce Diet has been awesome! Almost done with 3 Weeks to Shredded & my size 6 jeans are getting baggy! Started with size 8 being comfy! *-Jeanette*

Won 1st place at NAGA with The Dolce Diet! Weighed in at 156, came from 187 in just 18 days using 3 Weeks to Shredded! #livinglean *-Trey Manly*

I went from 215 lbs. to 188 lbs. in just over a month on 3 Weeks to Shredded. Using 3 Weeks to Shredded as my template, I started to change every part of my life, cleaning out the junk and replacing it with pure energy provided by the earth. My Dad went from 225 lbs. to 207 lbs. with 3 Weeks to Shredded! He is going for another 3 weeks to get to his goal of 185 lbs. #LivingLean *-Todd Harwood*

I was 192 lbs. 25 days ago - 154.9 today. Big thanks to 3 Weeks to Shredded. *-Eric Irvin*

@TheDolceDiet May 28 was 174 lbs. Today (June 21) before weigh ins was 154.5 lbs. #boom #livinglean #3w2s *-Salvador Woods*

Finally broke the 200 lbs. mark! So stoked! So far, down 31 lbs. #transformation #livinglean #3w2s #fitness #healthy @thedolcediet *-Justin L.*

LEAN AND MEAN!! 191-170 lbs. in three weeks all thanks to @thedolcediet #3w2s #dolceknows *-AJ Rodriguez*

@TheDolceDiet No supplement gave me better results than @LivingLeanBook and #3w2s. 216 lbs. to 164 lbs. in 4 months. *-Michael Santos*

A huge shout out to The Dolce Diet - changed my life! Wife and I are down a total of 134 lbs.! *-Justin Armstrong*

I'm down another 6 lbs. That's 11 lbs. in 7 days! *-Imran R.*

January 3 I was 364 lbs. Scale said 304.6 lbs. this morning March 28! #YodaWearsDolcePajamas *-Scott A. Schultz*

@TheDolceDiet Cheers, Mike! I've lost 20 kg. (45 lbs.) in 2.5 months. Went from a 42-inch waist to a 34-inch waist and not once felt like I was on a diet! *-Lynden Brench*

@TheDolceDiet Mike, big thanks for giving me my life back for my kids' sake. You pushed me from 263 lbs. (January) to 178 lbs. (June). 3 Weeks to Shredded ends tomorrow. Goal is 170 lbs. *-Shawn Brown*

My last weight cut - 16.7 lbs. in 22 days! Everything is possible with hard work and @TheDolceDiet *-Rickard Enbom*

@TheDolceDiet 3 Weeks to Shredded got me to 152 lbs. and 8-9% body fat for my 155 lbs. match! BOOM! #145Next *-Kyle Eberts*

Woke up on weight & ready for weigh-ins! Didn't even have to cut water weight. @TheDolceDiet is that good! Dropped 20 lbs. in eight weeks #mma *-Dan Perez*

Started at 215 lbs. back in April, now I'm 178! Thanks, Mike, for all the help and motivation. - *David W.*

When I started The Dolce Diet I was a 40-inch waist weighing in at 265 lbs. Six weeks later I'm a 36-inch waist and 50 lbs. lighter! *-Anderson W.*

After one week on this plan, I've dropped 6 lbs. SIX! For a woman that has been scale-conscious the past 5 years that was amazing to me. I can't thank Mike enough for creating this and putting it out there for all of us to experience for ourselves. I wish this was around years ago. *-Jennifer C.*

Working 60 hours a week but three weeks in on The Dolce Diet & I've lost 30 lbs. This is an awesome diet! Thank you so much for putting this out there for everyone! *-Nate F.*

This week I fit into a size 6 and literally cried. It was a huge moment in my life. For the past 6 years it's been a hassle getting ready in the mornings and having nothing fit and everything too tight. Barely squeezing into jeans made for one horrible day and frame of mind. But Monday morning when I fit into a pair of jeans I had from long ago, with nothing hanging over the sides, no jumping up and down to pull them up, just slipping into these cute pair of jeans that I've kept in the closet for motivation was a damn good feeling. *-Lyndsey F.*

The Dolce Diet is well worth it! I lost 10 lbs. in a week. This is the lightest I've been since high school!
-Justin A.

I've lost over 75 lbs. (and counting) as a student of Mike Dolce's. I have a second chance to live my life! *-Bonnie W.*

Fourteen pounds gone in 14 days on The Dolce Diet! *-Jason L.*

Mike and his Dolce Diet transformed me physically and mentally into who I am today. I started at 32.6 percent body fat & last tested at 8.7 percent. Thanks for everything Mike! *-Brian S.*

I've lost 45 lbs.! I'd recommend anyone buy The Dolce Diet.
-Craig L.

I'm down 25 lbs. in 2 months! People have seen my changes and are encouraged to begin their transformation. *-Mike P.*

---

219 lbs. to 193 lbs. in a month-and-a-half thanks to The Dolce Diet! *-Jake C.*

The book has worked wonders already! I dropped 15+ lbs. Thanks! *-Monroe D.*

I went from 220 lbs. to 180 in 1 month on The Dolce Diet.
-Mark A.

Just finished my first 21-day weight cut on The Dolce Diet, and I'm in the best shape of my life! Successfully cut from 185 lbs. to 168! Thanks for doin' whatchado! *-John P.*

Fifteen pounds lost in 21 days! The Dolce Diet included great results, improved energy levels, more efficient training sessions and clearer thinking. Thank you, Mike Dolce, for making permanent, positive changes to my life. *-Heather P.*

In two weeks I dropped 13 lbs. and my buddy has dropped 10 lbs. Things are looking good! Thanks! *-Andrew M.*

In 17 days I dropped over 18 lbs. I'm looking and feeling fantastic! *-Aaron R.*

I've been doing The Dolce Diet for almost 5 months, and I have lost a total of 40lbs. *-Mary*

I'm under 200 lbs. in a few weeks! I've lost just over 17 lbs. & I'm so excited about it. *-Aaron F.*

The Dolce Diet is killing me. In another two weeks I will be broke from having to replace all of my jeans and shorts with smaller sizes. I literally have lost a waist size in two weeks. Absolute truth. *-Wes H.*

Started The Dolce Diet at 209.8 lbs. It's Day 4 and I'm at 203.6 lbs.! *-Tom C.*

Eighty-pound loss mark today. The Dolce Diet and determination truly goes a long way. *-Allen C.*

All testimonials from emailed correspondence, Facebook, Twitter or Instagram.

Part 1

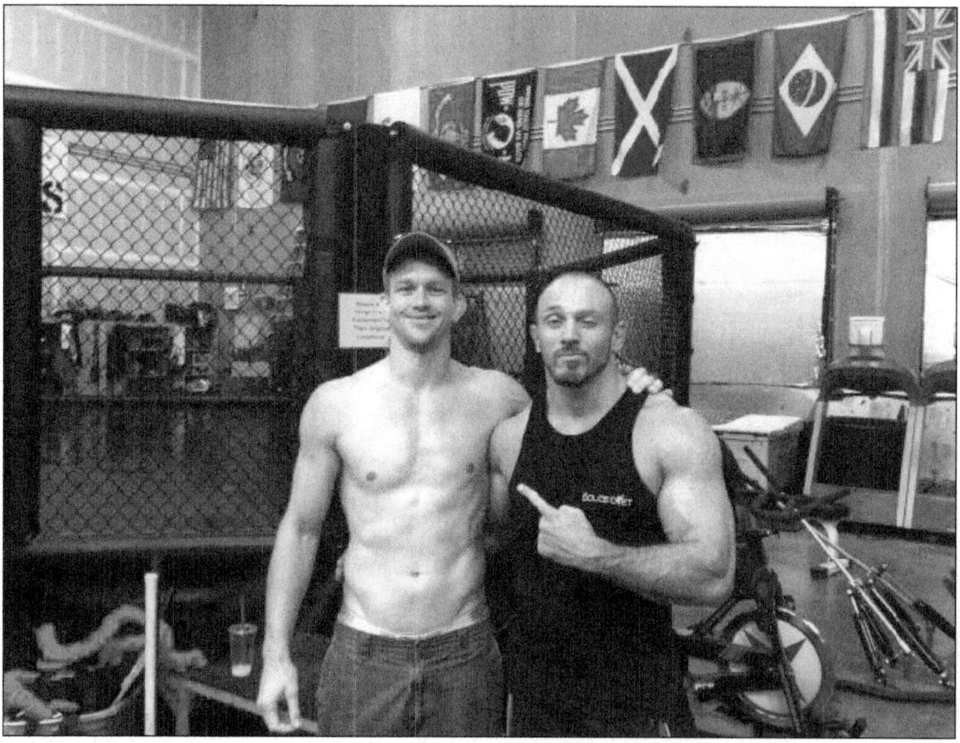

UFC Welterweight Mike "Quicksand" Pyle wraps up another training session leading up to his bout with Rick Story at UFC 160 on May 25, 2013.

DOLCE DIET PRINCIPLES

> ***"The underlying principles of strategy are enduring, regardless of technology or the pace of change."*** *~Michael Porter*

Whether you're a professional mixed martial artist, a CEO, a new mom, or an ultra-marathon runner, the Dolce Diet Principles below apply to every BODY! They are evergreen, no matter how the world around us changes. Stick to these principles, and you will always know the answer to what some may think is the most difficult question in the world: "What's for dinner?"

1. Earth-Grown Nutrients

This is food that comes organically from this planet, untouched by man. Science and evolution have shown this class of food is most readily absorbed, digested and utilized with maximum nutrition and minimum calories. Regardless of what you see on TV, man "and his marketing machines" have not, will not and cannot replace the optimal nutrition of Earth-grown nutrients. Categorically, when an athlete converts to The Dolce Diet, they immediately throw out the pills, powders and potions and adopt a diet consisting solely of Earth-grown nutrients. The results have been astounding and are proven nearly every weekend on TV. If this method did not work, neither would I.

2. Eat Every 2 To 4 Hours.

In my research - both scientific and practical - the vast majority of the human species performs at greater levels more consistently when eating every 2 to 4 hours based upon what we just did and what we are about to do. There are many reasons for this.

The top 3 being:

a) Improved metabolism, or the rate at which we process food to create energy.
b) Insulin sensitivity - if off-balance, it can affect the way we digest carbohydrates and absorb nutrients.
c) Post exercise recovery, a topic of primary importance to those reading this book.

There are popular fad diets that make their way through pop culture from time to time, based upon fasting or juicing or cleansing or eliminating specific food groups or various combinations of each. The benefit of these programs are traditionally short-lived and counterproductive in the long term. If any of these worked as well as eating sensible, high nutrition meals at even intervals, would it not make sense for my multimillion dollar athletes to follow suit? Again, I would be out of work.

3. Eat Until Satisfied Not Until Full.
The biggest problem with frequent feedings is lack of control over quantity and quality of nutrients consumed. As a rule, when we eat we should feel energized and revitalized. I ask my athletes to ask themselves at the conclusion of each meal, "Can I go for a 45-minute jog right now?" If the answer is "No," you've eaten incorrectly. There is no need to gorge yourself at any meal when you know you can eat again within 2 to 4 hours.

By overstuffing our digestive tract, we become less efficient at metabolizing those nutrients. Our metabolism slows down and we become sluggish. Picture a locomotive steaming down the tracks. The engineer must shovel coal at even intervals in manageable amounts to keep the engine burning bright and hot. Put too much coal in and the flame goes out, the engine stops. Put too little coal in, again the flame is extinguished and the engine stops. The key here is constant feedings in a quantity that is easy to digest.

4. Optimal Hydration

Water has sustained all of life on this planet since the dawn of time - H2O is the elixir of life. Not high fructose corn syrup. By water, I mean purified water. Not soda, processed juices, sports beverages, or electrolyte-enhanced concoctions made for babies.

Real water is essential for the cellular function of every biological process, including digestion, muscular contraction, cognitive function - essentially LIFE! Water is second only to oxygen on the list of human survival with food coming in at a distant third place.

As a rule, a human being can survive 2 minutes without oxygen, 2 days without water and 2 weeks without food. Unfortunately, too many of us neglect the importance of water. When it comes to cutting weight, water is everything.

5. Stay Accountable.

There are a million reasons to blow your diet, and one reason to stick to it. Your goals. These 5 principles above should be your mantra.

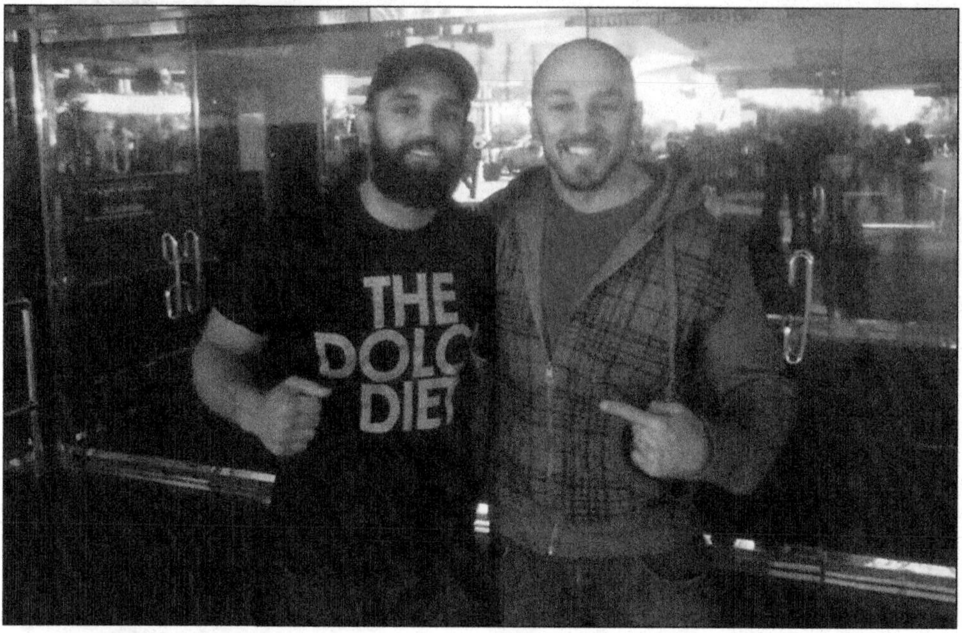

Longtime Dolce Diet client Johny Hendricks smiles on the eve of his devastating first-round knockout of John Fitch.

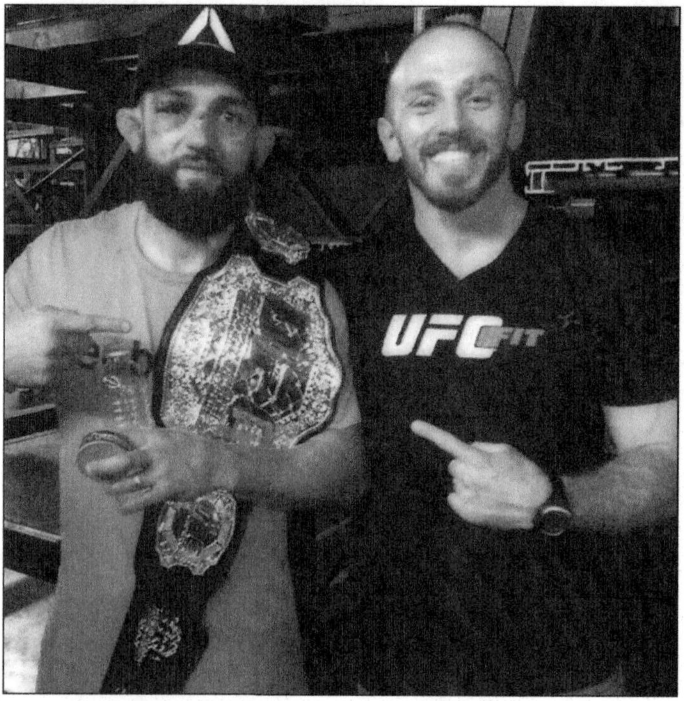

Six fights later, Johny Hendricks captures the UFC Welterweight world title.

THE IMPORTANCE OF GOALS

Just the word GOAL invokes a destination. Whether it be an end zone, a mountain top or a smaller waist size, we all know what a goal should be. The problem I often come across is that people have loose goals. They kid themselves by pretending to have set a goal, when really they just have a wish. "I want to lose weight," is the most common but often goes no further than that statement.

When confronted with this person I always ask, "How much exactly? What deadline have you set? Did you create action steps to get there?" Very rarely is my first question answered and almost never are my second two even considered.

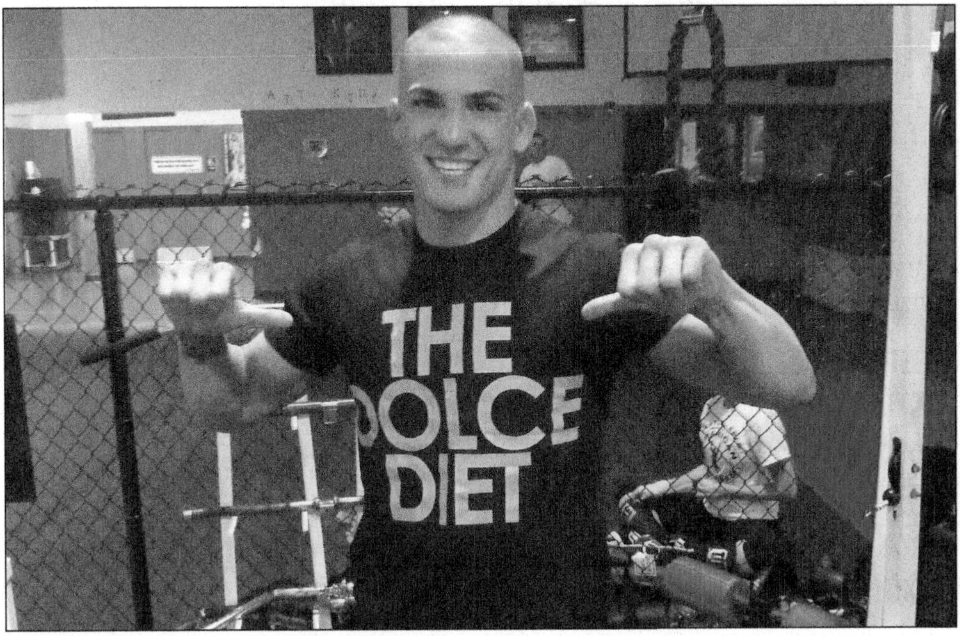

Undefeated professional Mirsad Bektic proudly represents The Dolce Diet prior to his victorious UFC debut in 2014.

This is when I switch into COACH MODE and make sure my friend has a clearly defined plan before walking away.

This can sometimes be inconvenient because I am often recognized as being "that diet guy" in coffee shops, gyms, malls and for some reason ALWAYS at the movie theatre. My wife usually looks at me with a smile, knowing we are now going to miss the opening credits while I attempt to change the course of my new friend's life.

"Begin TODAY! There is no better time like the present. Don't push it off until Monday."

STEP 1
Set a clearly defined goal.
"I WILL (not want to) lose 40 lbs."
Now you have a very clear picture of your exact destination. There is no confusion here.

STEP 2
"I WILL lose 40 lbs. in 120 days."
Now you have a specific timeline. No more circling the drain, waiting to begin. The clock is now ticking.

STEP 3
"I WILL lose 40 lbs. in 120 days by following these ACTION STEPS."

ACTION STEP 1: Using The Dolce Diet principles I will create my own lifestyle approach to weight loss using the principles, recipes and exercise programs that Mike has already laid out, most suited to my own ability, goals and medical background.

ACTION STEP 2: Be consistent. For the next 120 days (and rest of my life) I will dedicate myself to achieving this goal and hold myself 100 percent accountable. Regardless of what unexpected trial or tribulation may come up in my life, I will continue on with my goal until I have found success.

ACTION STEP 3: Create a support system. This may be your family, friends, team, coworkers or online community. I have started such a community at MYDolceDiet.com for all of us to support, motivate and inspire each other as we all travel toward our own unique goals. Pro-athletes, bikini models, lawyers, students, moms, law enforcement professionals and many others are members and the community is thriving! Create your own community or join ours.

ACTION STEP 4: Begin TODAY! There is no better time like the present. Don't push it off until Monday. Start now, as best you can, and continue making improvements the first few days. It doesn't matter if you haven't gone grocery shopping yet, or have a trip scheduled. Begin moving toward your goal immediately and constantly work to improve your situation as you go. Start NOW!

ACTION STEP 5: I also instruct my students to sit down with a notebook they have purchased specifically for this project and write down everything - your goals, a more complete version of these steps with greater detail as it relates to your specific situation, your daily bodyweight, progress at the gym, frustrations, successes and so on. This book becomes your own training partner, support system, cherished friend and annoying cheerleader reminding you of how far you have come.

The Action Steps above are general but apply to each of you. Ultimately, you know everything I have said above. I did not break new ground here and that was not my intention.

My GOAL here was to get you accountable and for you to START RIGHT NOW!

"Set higher standards for your own performance than anyone else around you, and your only competition will be with yourself." ~Rick Pitino

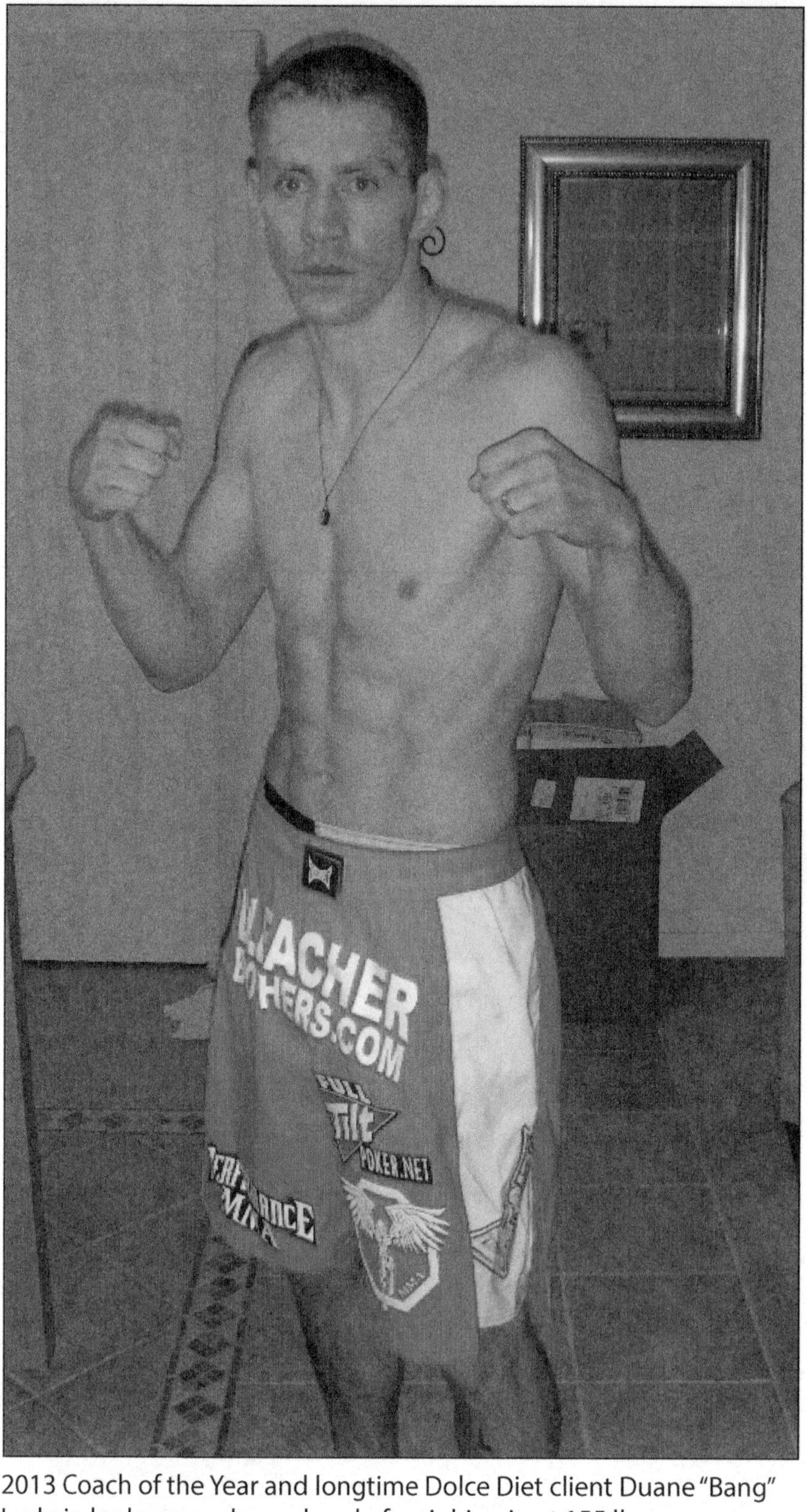

2013 Coach of the Year and longtime Dolce Diet client Duane "Bang" Ludwig looks razor sharp ahead of weighing in at 155 lbs.

21 DAYS, 21 GOALS

> ***"We first make our habits, and then our habits make us."*** *-John Dryden*

Now you know you want to make a change. The first step is to break current habits that are moving you away from your goals and create new habits that will move you closer.

Over the next 3 weeks, we will focus on transitioning your current set of habits to a more productive set of habits. Your progress will depend largely on your ability to change, to be flexible, and to be open minded, to let go and grab hold at exactly the same time.

Over the next 21 days, you will set 21 small goals. Make them simple but meaningful. Find a piece of paper and a pen. Write down tomorrow's goal. You will achieve that one small goal tomorrow. Tomorrow night you will set the next day's goal.

Mine might look like this:

03/11/07 Run 5 miles.
This is a good, simple goal for me, because I typically run 4 miles each day. Adding 1 extra mile will not kill me, yet it will extend my ability.

03/12/07 Eat breakfast with my wife.
- My wife and I have busy schedules and don't eat breakfast together enough.

Tomorrow, I will wake up with her and cook us breakfast while she "does her thing."

03/13/07 Be 10 minutes early to each practice and shadowbox.

- I have 3 practices tomorrow. An extra 30 minutes of shadowboxing is basically another workout in itself. And, at 10 minute increments, my day won't be affected.

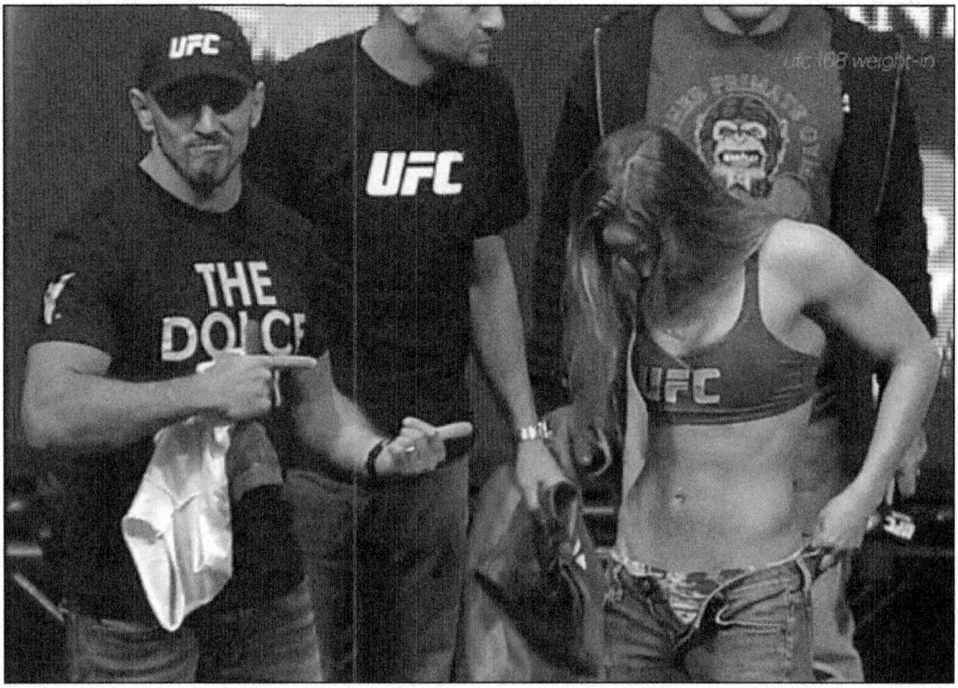

"Rowdy" Ronda Rousey gets ready to weigh in for her title defense against Miesha "Cupcake" Tate at UFC 168. Rousey defeated Tate with a third-round armbar.

"Limits are self imposed. But there are no limits to human energy nor the goals you can achieve."

~Mike Shanahan

GOALS WORKSHEET

Do not skip this chapter! This is where you set your goals for the first 3 weeks of this program. After that, you should set new goals in your own private notebook.

This is what my athletes do. This is what the multimillion-dollar CEOs who hire me do. The one thing we all have in common is that we set daily goals to ensure our progress. Just like the captain of a ship constantly needs to check his compass, so must you constantly set and evaluate new goals!

Start writing!

WEEK 1

WEEK 2

WEEK 3

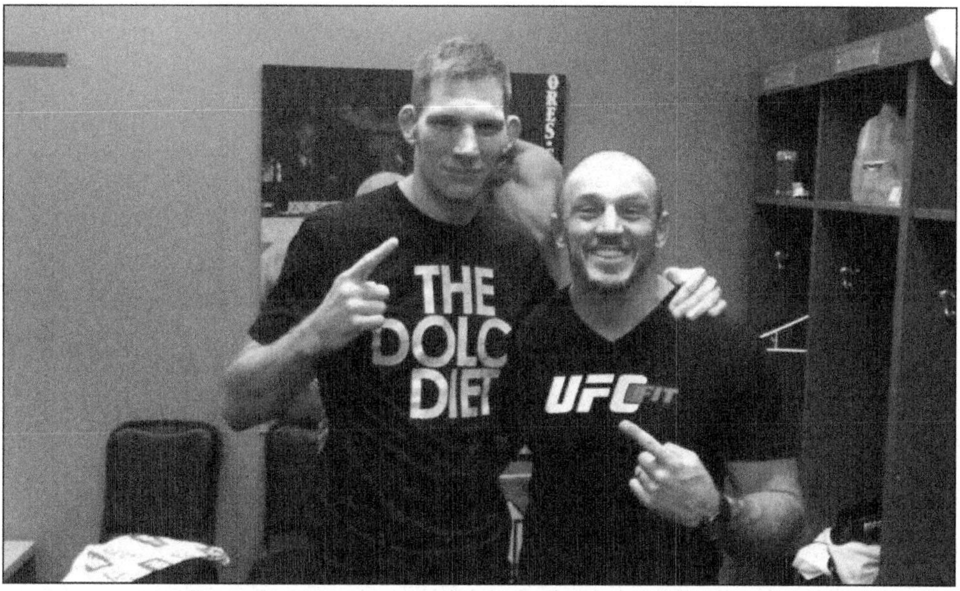

Great Britain's own Luke Barnatt became a Dolce Diet athlete during season 17 of The Ultimate Fighter. Luke has become one of the UFC's fastest rising stars.

TODD HARWOOD

Starting weight: 215 lbs. • Ending weight: 187 lbs.

As of March 2013 it has been 2 solid years since I changed my lifestyle and started living lean.

I started at 215 lbs. After my first round of 3 Weeks to Shredded, commonly known in social media as 3W2S, I dropped 28 lbs. and have not looked back. I am at, and have constantly remained at, 187 lbs. plus or minus a few lbs.

No, it has not been easy; we all have our peaks and valleys. I never expected it to be easy. After all, real life is not like some commercial where you sprinkle some powder on your chili dog and everything turns out all right. Nothing valuable comes easy.

This lifestyle requires you to be accountable to yourself, become reliant upon yourself, and make choices and live with the consequences of those choices - the good ones and the bad. It requires that you self govern and motivate yourself. See a theme here? This is about you and what you do; it has no chance of getting done otherwise.

Self-motivation is a huge aspect of this lifestyle, but we all get down on ourselves at times and need help. This is where the masterful Mike Dolce steps in. Listen and re-listen to his podcasts. It is like having him over your shoulder coaching you anytime, anywhere through your ear buds.

*Use MyDolceDiet.com and The Dolce Diet Facebook page; ask questions, start discussions. You get no answer right away? Hit Twitter - if Mike doesn't answer himself (which is crazy; I think he has clones of himself) then #hashtag that ****ing tweet! Get with it! #3W2S #LivingLean #TheDolceDiet #LivingLeanCookBook #EarthGrownNutrients*

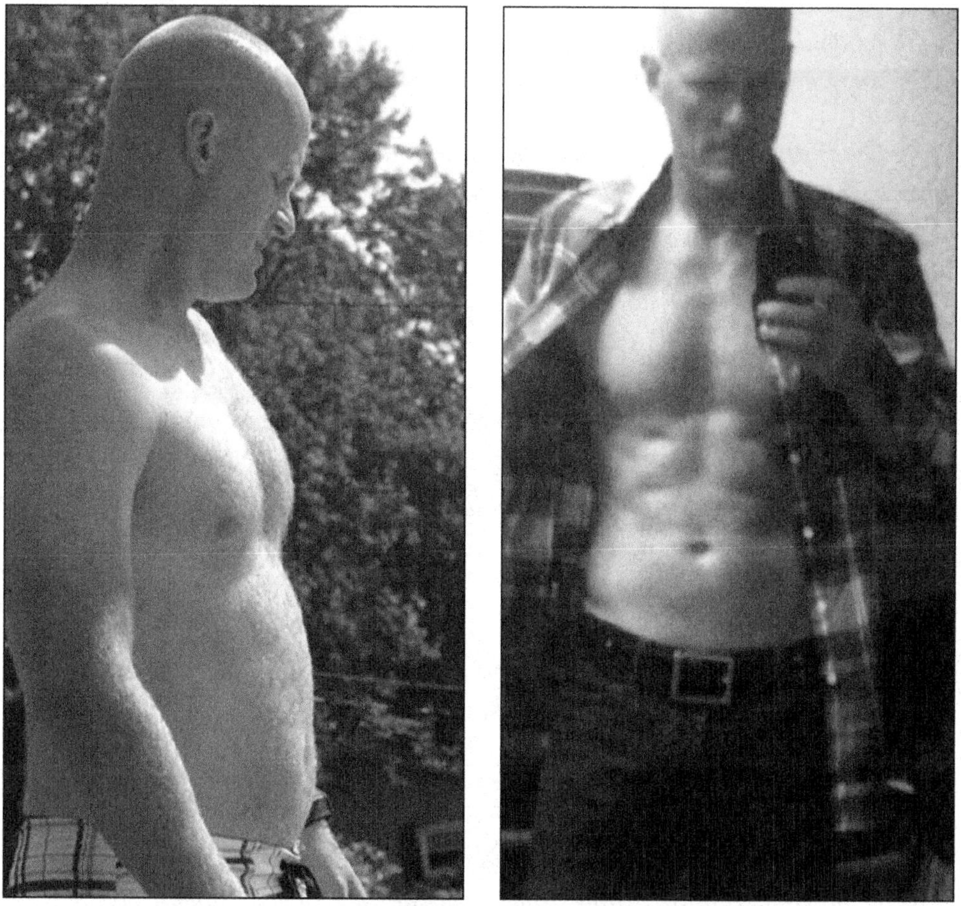

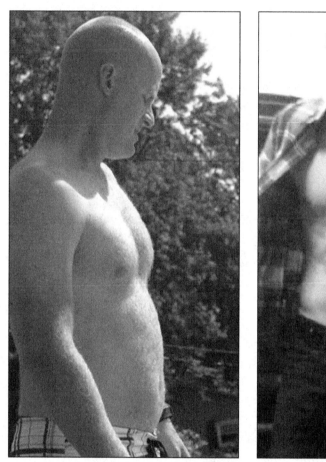

Todd Harwood before The Dolce Diet at 215 lbs. and after at 187 lbs.

#HelpMeDolce (LOL) Somebody in this Living Lean Community will see it and get back to you. Use this team as a motivational tool.

Mike Dolce and Brandy Dolce are like your Training Camp coaches, except this isn't a 6-week or 12-week camp; this is for life! Don't give up – don't give in. Use the resources available to your advantage. Make friends, follow, check @TheDolceDiet's favorites, fill up your favorites with other people's inspiring tweets and success stories, and go back and use those to motivate you. It works! I do it.

I have a vacation to Hawaii coming up. I leave April 23 to paradise and I plan on being half naked about 98.9 percent of the time I am there. I am going to be surfing, swimming, paddle boarding, hiking, kayaking. I am going to squeeze every ounce of health and vitality that I have been blessed with, count on it. Like I said, I am also going to be half naked, constantly – so I start another round of 3 Weeks to Shredded on April 1. I have already marked my calendar with my GOAL that by the weekend of April 20, I will be a lean, mean, washboard-abs machine!

Mike doesn't type and talk until he is blue in the face for us to not take heed. He does it so we will set goals and do our very best to reach those goals. I consider Mike and his team to be my coaches, and coaches with this high level of passion and this much availability come around maybe once in a lifetime. I plan on reaping the blessings that come with their dedication and their want for me to succeed. I will not squander this opportunity.

I hope this encourages you to set your own personal goals and reach the high level of health and vitality that we are all capable of.

"Most of the shadows of this life are caused by our standing in our own sunshine."
~Ralph Waldo Emerson

WEIGHT CUT OR WEIGHT LOSS? WHAT'S THE DIFFERENCE?

I recently received a message from a person who is morbidly obese and is looking to make "a weight cut" – of 100 lbs. Let's be clear. This is not a weight cut. This is weight loss.

The increased popularity of Mixed Martial Arts has the words "weight cut" falling off people's lips like it's a trend. In fact, the weight-cut process walks a very precise, often dangerous line between what is healthy and what is hapless, and should not be taken lightly – pun definitely intended! I define a weight cut as a temporary reduction of the body's water volume. Keyword here? TEMPORARY!

A weight cut is something an athlete does for a weight-class delineated competition. This athlete is typically already at a healthy bodyweight with an ideal ratio of lean mass to body fat while training for his or her competition. Weight loss is something most people pursue in an effort to become healthier, leaner and to create the ability to live a more vibrant, fuller life. Weight loss focuses on the elimination of non-functional weight – the weight that is bogging you down and getting you nowhere! It interferes with our function as a healthy and thriving individual.

FUNCTIONAL VS. NON-FUNCTIONAL WEIGHT

If you weigh 195 lbs. at 20 percent body fat, you have 39 lbs. of body fat and 156 lbs. of muscle, bones, skin and organs, or functional weight.

At 20 percent body fat, you have no idea what your abs look like and are at a high risk factor for heart disease, diabetes and early death.

Now, if you weigh 195 lbs. at 10 percent body fat, you look absolutely amazing. You only have 19.5 lbs. of nonfunctional weight, most of which is insulation from the environment, protects your joints and ligaments and

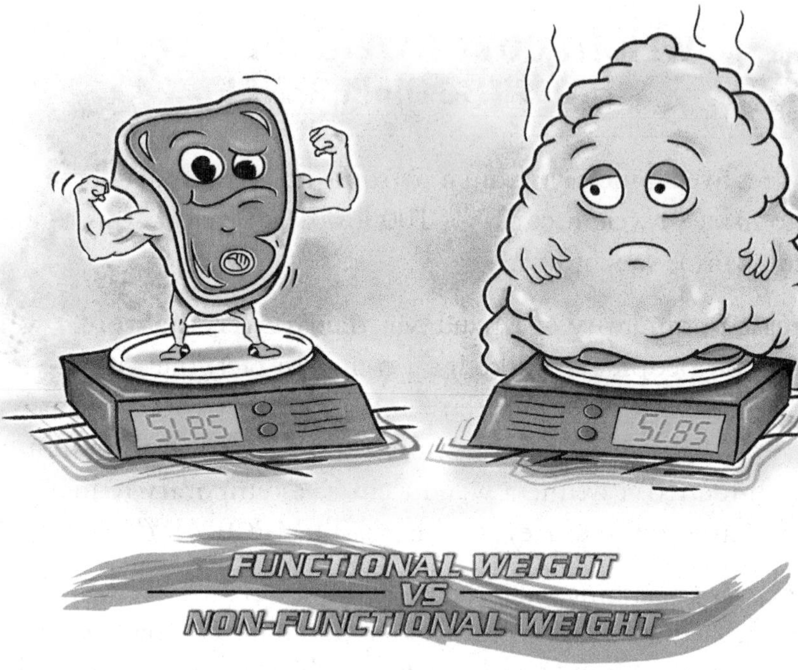

serves as readily usable energy. You also have 175.5 lbs. of functional bodyweight, which is quite a lot compared to the chubbier version of yourself.

How different is 20 lbs. of muscle? I like to tell people to picture a 16 oz. steak sitting on your dinner plate. Now multiply that by 20 and stick them all over your body like Lady Gaga's meat dress. Yes, 20 lbs. of lean muscle is quite substantial. What does 20 lbs. of body fat look like? A great visual would be to fill up 2 entire gallon milk jugs of butter and cottage cheese, plus a 2 liter soda bottle of the same and pour it in a backpack, or better yet a REALLY BIG fanny pack sloshing around your hips! How would it feel slugging around that load of lard?

For the average healthy adult male, we should maintain body-fat levels at approximately 10 percent. I don't care if you are happy being 12 percent or you say, "I'm too old to be lower than 15 percent" - that is your preference. You can drive around in an '89 Honda Accord with low miles, but have you seen that new Ferrari?!

Professional male athletes should be around 7 percent body fat for competition purposes. With my athletes, I make sure they are at 7 percent body fat 3 weeks before competition so we can increase their calories as competition nears. In essence, we feed them onto the scale.

The last couple of lbs. (or dozen lbs. depending on the athlete) is simply a matter of adjusting electrolytes, stimulating their metabolism and managing their digestive environment. A much simpler way of putting this is to feed them familiar, nutrient dense, easy to absorb foods, at even intervals but not so much to slow digestion, in fact, just enough to speed it up. Ladies, you should aim for 20 percent body fat as your daily walk around weight and closer to 16 percent for most higher levels of athletics. This means the average 130 lb. woman at 20 percent body fat would hold 26 lbs. of non-functional body fat and 104 lbs. of functional lean mass weight.

That same female, if she were a competitive athlete, would best be suited in the vicinity of 16 percent body fat, would carry 20.8 lbs. of non-functional body fat and 109.2 lbs. of functional lean mass weight.

WHAT DOES ALL THIS MEAN FOR THE AVERAGE INDIVIDUAL?
It means, do you really want to look your best or are you going to be happy with just looking a little better, which is fine but it is well below your potential.

Let's face it, life is much more enjoyable with your clothes off! Before you drag this book into the gutter, I'm referring to the confidence you feel when you walk into a room with a tight waistline hidden behind your little black dress or formfitting suit.

Who doesn't want to be the first one in the pool with zero reservations about pulling off your shirt?

Why wouldn't you want to keep the lights on when you are, umm, getting undressed? The point is, aim for your best, enjoy where you are but always strive to do better.

Take it from me. I used to weigh 280 lbs. while training as a power lifter. This was my choice, and even though my ego was constantly gratified with bigger numbers on the barbell and trophies on my mantle, I hated the feeling of my belly sitting on my belt as I drove in my truck. Once I decided to change my goals and purse a longevity-based lifestyle, I immediately began to love myself. I had enormous energy, a much improved sense of self and also the confidence of setting a goal and seeing it all the way through to the end.

On the opposite page is a picture of the new me at 180 lbs. at 5 percent body fat, and the old me, who once weighed 280 lbs. at 22 percent body fat!

Many of us, myself included, must be focused on fat loss and functional bodyweight. Not "cutting weight."

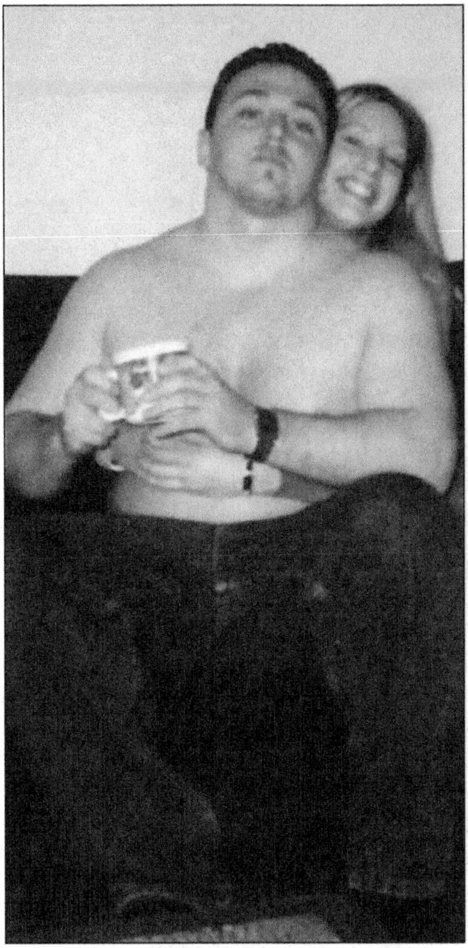

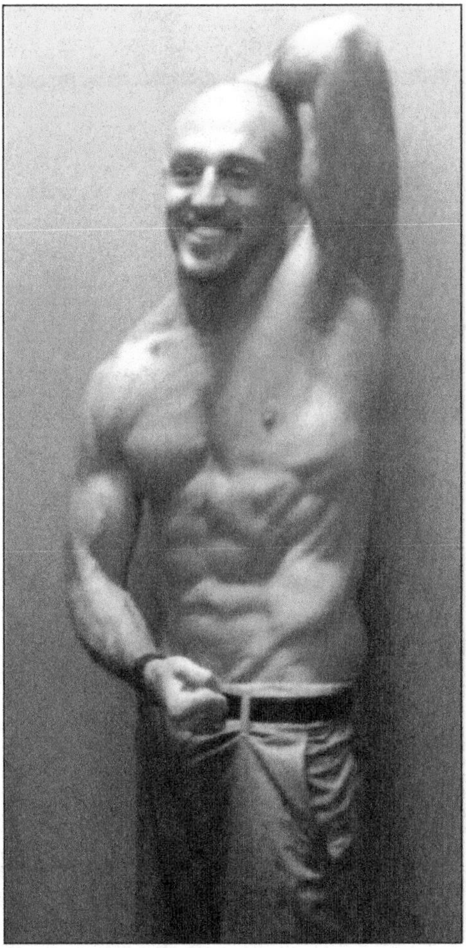

The proof is in the picture. The old Mike Dolce at 22 percent body fat and the new Mike Dolce at 5 percent body fat.

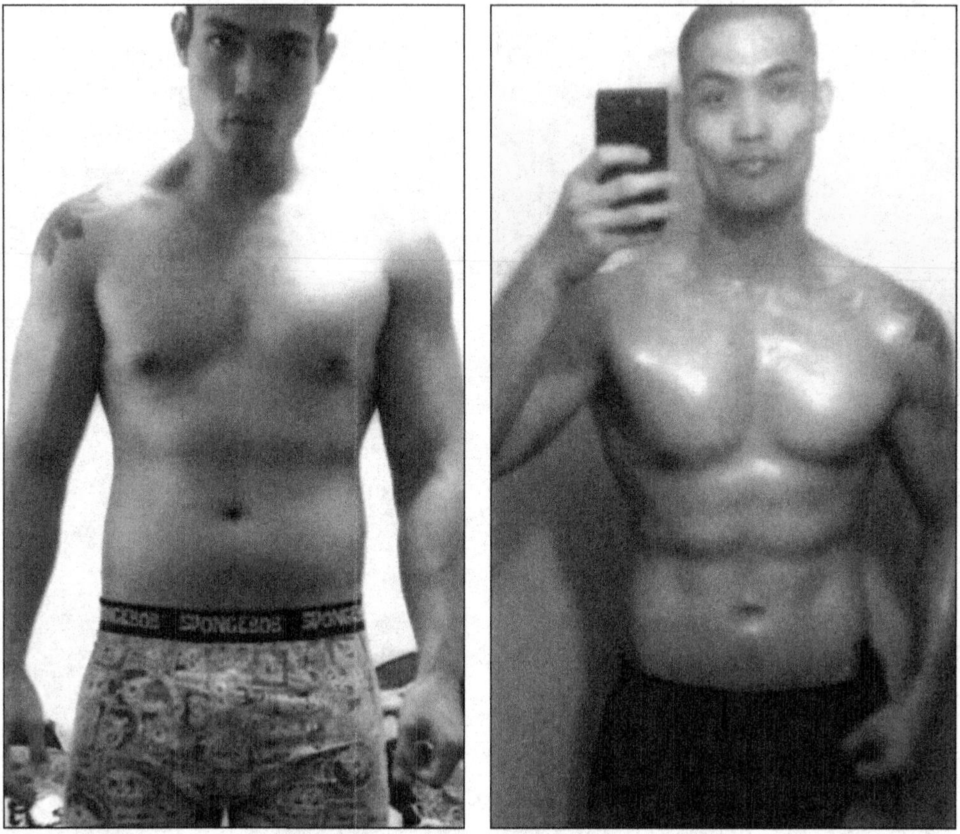

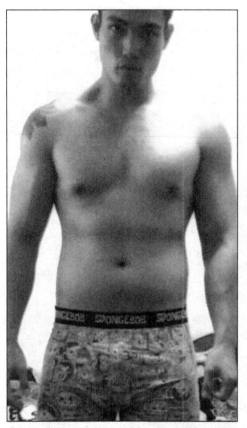

Michael Santos before The Dolce Diet at 216 lbs. and after at 164 lbs.

MICHAEL SANTOS

Starting weight: 216 lbs. • Ending weight: 164 lbs.

Throughout my life, I have always struggled with weight. After joining the gym, I began putting on muscle weight, yet fat continued to sit in front of it. I knew that my diet was preventing me from getting the body I want.

Being a big fan of MMA, I constantly heard about The Dolce Diet so I decided to research it. After reading the testimonials, I decided my goal was to be one of these people. I ordered 3 Weeks to Shredded and Living Lean right away.

My starting weight was 216 lbs. at 21 percent body fat. I started 3 Weeks to Shredded and followed it religiously. After three weeks, I went down to 174 lbs.

After finishing, I continued with Living Lean. Because of this book, I was able to continue my transformation by continually losing body fat while increasing my muscle mass.

Now I'm proudly walking around at 164 lbs. at 9.3 percent body fat and in the best shape of my life. The Dolce Diet changed my body more in 4 months than all the diet and workout supplements have done combined.

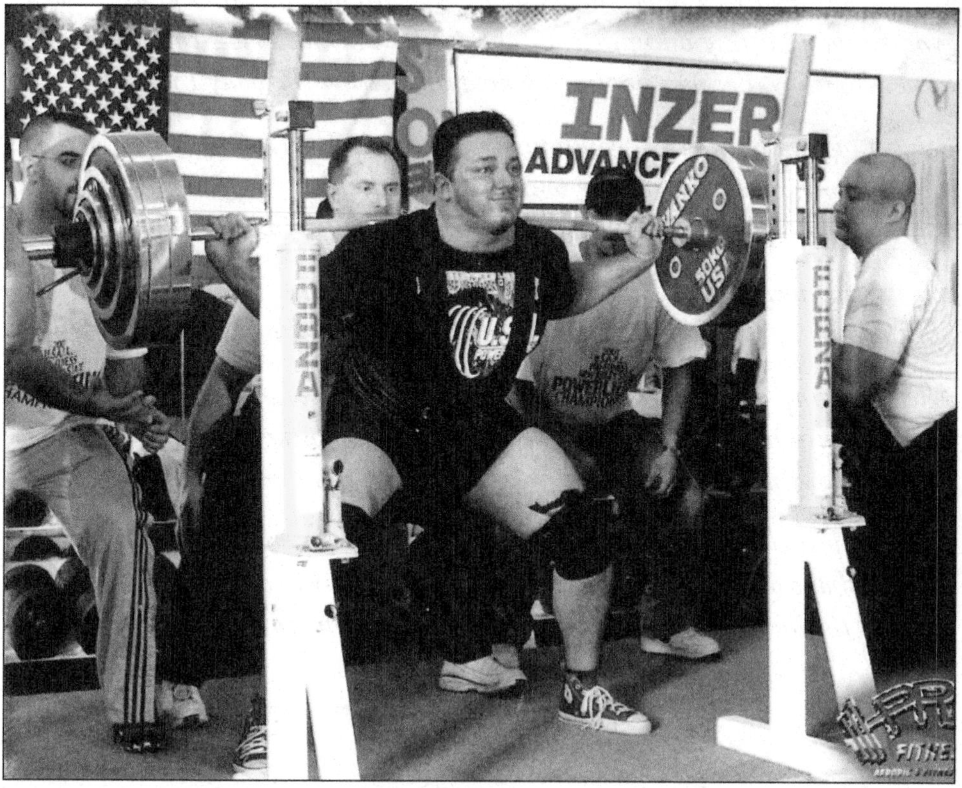

Mike Dolce back in his powerlifting days, weighing 280 lbs.

SO YOU WANT TO CUT WEIGHT - GETTING STARTED

Motivation is a funny thing, and most of the time, the joke is on us because many think motivation is pulled from external sources. It's not. It's harnessed from within. It stems from our passion, what we want, our goals, the way we imagine life could and should be. Ironically, most people blame others when they don't get what they want. Why? I'm not sure. Maybe because it wasn't handed to them in pretty gift wrap with a giant red bow.

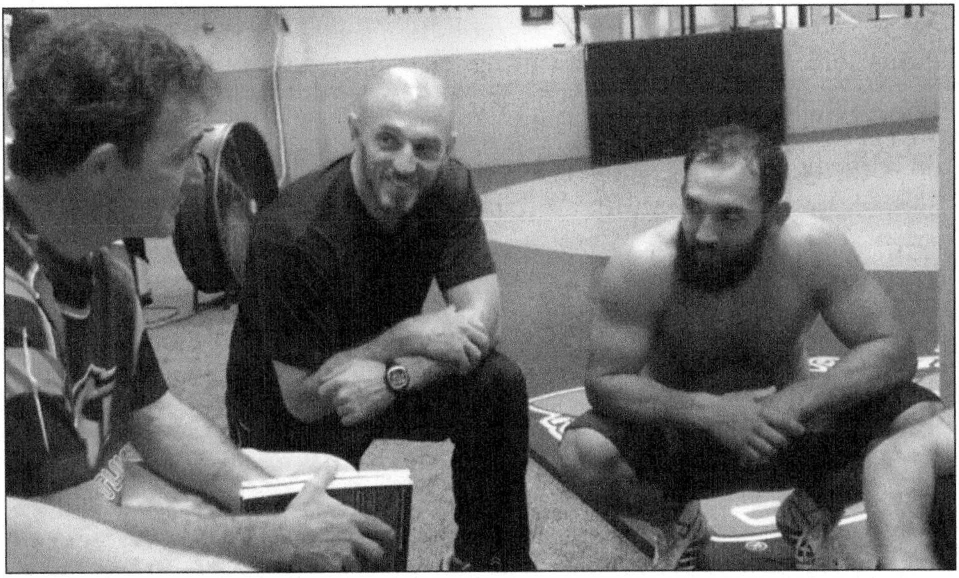

(From left) Oklahoma State head wrestling coach John Smith, Mike Dolce, and UFC welterweight champion Johny "Bigg Rigg" Hendricks.

For the next 3 weeks, you must be accountable to this program. Within the first few days, you will begin to feel the positive effects of this lifestyle. We must keep that momentum going and establish lifelong habits. It will take a few days to get in the rhythm. Once you have a rhythm, you will start to see results.

As the results come, your body may begin to resist in various ways, your mind may play tricks on you and this is where your challenge lies. The first hurdle. You will overcome that hurdle and you will break through to a whole new level of health.

Your goals are YOURS. Never allow the actions of others to detract from your goals. And NEVER piggyback your wants and needs on someone else's. If they lose focus, you need to keep yours. If they can't stay the course, you must keep hacking through the jungle to your own destination. The prize is there waiting for you to raise it high above your head. And oh, what a feeling that will be!

You've likely heard this quote often attributed to Ghandi. "Be the change you wish to see in the world." What he actually said was much, much wiser.

> ***"If we could change ourselves, the tendencies in the world would also change. As a man changes his own nature, so does the attitude of the world change towards him. ... We need not wait to see what others do."** ~Muhatma Ghandi*

Do not wait for others to begin your journey to greatness. Within your passion, you will find your fire and you'll use it to blast away all obstacles, excuses, naysayers and the like. Failure is only failure if you allow it to be. There is no such word in my vocabulary. Now it's your turn to eradicate all doubt. Close your eyes, grasp your inner fire, and torch the word "failure" to ashes.

FRASER OPIE

Starting weight: 230 lbs. • Ending weight: 184 lbs.

It took 3.5 weeks to go from 230 lbs. to 202 lbs. I maintained 202 lbs. for 5 days, then cut the other 18 lbs. in 24 hours through a salt bath.

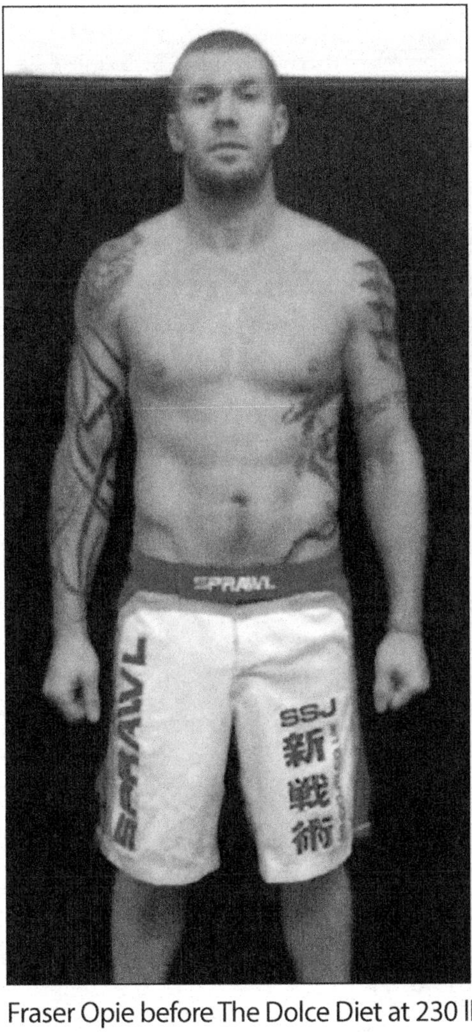

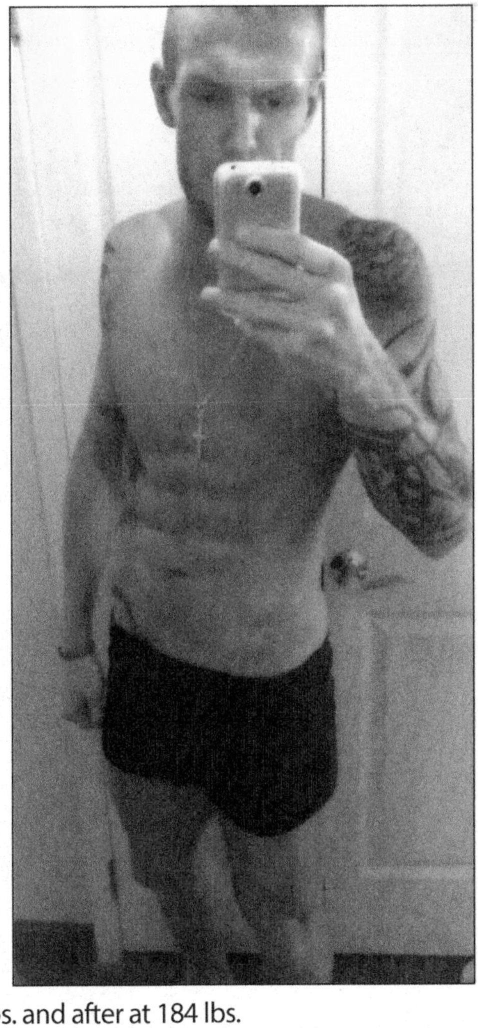

Fraser Opie before The Dolce Diet at 230 lbs. and after at 184 lbs.

"Build for your team a feeling of oneness, of dependence on one another and of strength to be derived by unity."
-Vince Lombardi

A LOOK INSIDE THE WEIGHT CUT

The best possible way to cut weight is to PLAN for it and START as soon as you're notified of the date of competition.

All too often we hear the horror stories of a poorly planned weight cut.

Vomiting.

Loss of sight.

Loss of hearing.

Loss of consciousness.

Even at the highest level of sport, athletes still miss weight and under-perform during competition as a result of difficulties endured during the final week of preparation. Unfortunately, during the most crucial time of the training camp, most fighters forget about the opponent on Saturday night and blindly scramble to figure out how to win the battle with the scale just 24 hours earlier. The old stigma of an exhausted athlete wrapped in plastic bags doing jumping jacks in a 180 degree Fahrenheit sauna is a reality that still holds true for many professionals.

The time you spend reading this just may save you from such a fate. In my experience, the healthier the athlete, the better his performance. Don't give me that crap about mental toughness and how champions have to overcome adversity as a means to justify an archaic and uninformed peaking plan. Those statements are easy to say when you are the one standing outside the sauna leaning on the door while the athlete cooks inside contemplating death.

I have spoken with too many athletes who share the same stories about passing out and wondering how they will survive the weight-cut process. The extreme levels of anxiety induced are the polar opposite of the mental state that will cultivate a career defining performance.

This is why I make safeguarding the health of my athlete the primary goal and making weight the secondary goal.

With this approach, the weight cut is easy because the athlete is fully nourished and hydrated, affording him the strength and nutrient reserves to go through the process of flushing fluids from his system.

This process does not start during fight week. It should start many years earlier with an adherence to a well-balanced diet of Earth-grown nutrients. For now, we are going to talk about fight week.

Fight week officially begins on Tuesday for professional mixed martial arts athletes. Each athlete and their team are flown to the site of the fight. The athlete is taken directly from the airport to the promoter's offices and immediately put on the scale. Once we register our weight on the official scale, we then weigh the athlete on our own personal scale to ensure we are calibrated.

It is not unusual for my athlete to weigh approximately 20 lbs. over the class limit, fully fed, hydrated and full of energy. We then check into our hotel rooms and begin the process of planning out the week. At the world-class MMA level, there are many obligations associated with fight week, such as photo shoots, interviews and personal appearances. Once we are handed the schedule, every moment of the day is planned, including the time we wake, eat and sweat.

Many athletes stop eating right about this time because that is the only way they know. They also stop drinking, reaching a dehydrated state many days before weigh-ins. At this point, the athlete already is in a weakened state. Combine this with grueling workouts in hot rooms while wrapped in a plastic sauna suit, and follow it by sessions in the sauna or hot tub, all on 0 calories, 2 to 3 times daily for several days and you have what constitutes a typical weight cut for many of the best athletes in the world.

That doesn't exactly sound like the most effective method for one to compete at 100 percent of his ability on Saturday night, does it?
If you have trained properly in the 6 to 8 weeks prior to the fight and followed an intelligent diet of Earth-grown nutrients in stable amounts and regular portions throughout the day, you should be quite lean - optimally between 7 to 10 percent body fat for male combat athletes (16 to 20 percent body fat for females).

Loss of body fat is no longer the goal 10 to 14 days before the fight. Now it is mostly a matter of water reduction - not reduction in consumption. More on this later.

Many athletes drop their water consumption way too soon, which may lead to a lighter scale weight, but the athlete also is putting his health at risk…not to mention he's weakening his strength and energy stores for the fight he's hoping to win just 24 hours later.

My methods suggest eating enough to maintain an athlete's primary needs for health while minimizing calorie expenditure. This allows him to function on fewer calories than his body is accustomed to while leading to a dramatic, temporary drop in bodyweight.

We also increase the amount of water consumed on a daily basis. This not only hydrates the body but keeps the stress reflex from slowing down the release of water.

Many athletes are accustomed to working off the weight, usually with 3 to 5 rounds of mitt work and 3 to 5 rounds of grappling. Keep in mind 3 to 5 rounds is the athlete's goal, which he usually fails to meet because he passed out. I once saw an athlete train this way for 55 painful minutes and lose only 3.5 lbs. The next night, at my suggestion, he lost 8 lbs. in 40 minutes hanging out with me in the hot tub, feeling great the entire time.

There certainly are many effective methods of reducing one's weight before competition, but suffering is not one of them.

My athletes eat breakfast every morning during fight week, and it isn't just any breakfast; it is a feast! They will also eat 3 snacks, as well as a lunch and dinner. You can probably picture a grizzled veteran's look of disbelief when I first break down the general plan for fight week. Especially one who's endured years of painful and torturous weight cuts. But, as the weeks move forward, they cringe when they recall the old way they used to do it and revel in how enjoyable the process becomes now that they can eat.

All of our meal decisions are made in the moment, based upon the feedback with which we are presented. For example, if the athlete has media obligations between noon and 4pm and will be on his feet answering questions for most of that time, he will need considerably more calories than if he were laying around his hotel room playing video games. There is no perfect process, and the athlete is the boss. He is the one who has to step on the scale and then step into competition the next night. We, as coaches, are there to assist and support the athlete's goals, while always protecting his health.

Just like the captain of a ship navigating precious cargo through treacherous waters, a good coach must keep his hands on the wheel and continually update his course based upon what lays in front of him.

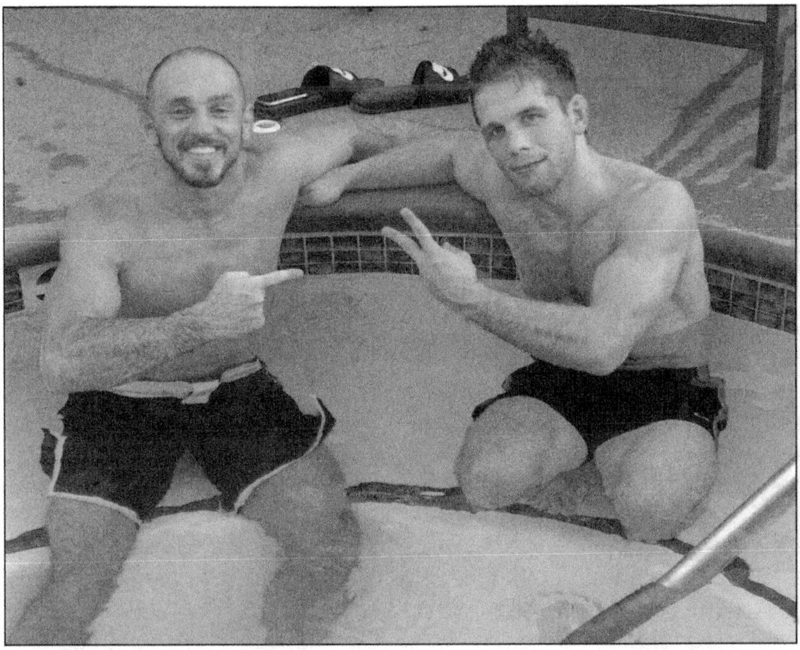

Nik Lentz relaxes through a weight cut using The Dolce Step Method.

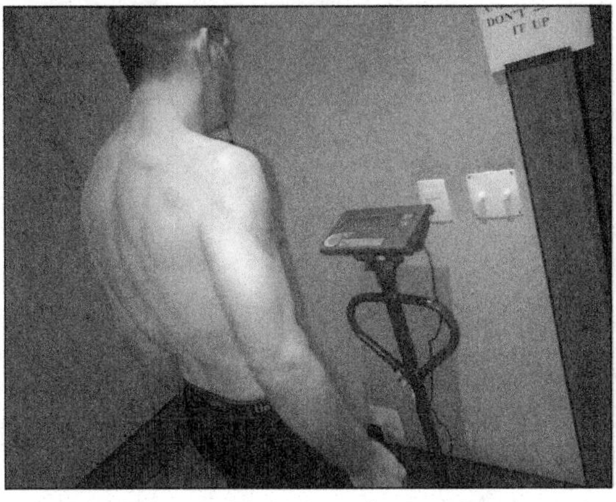

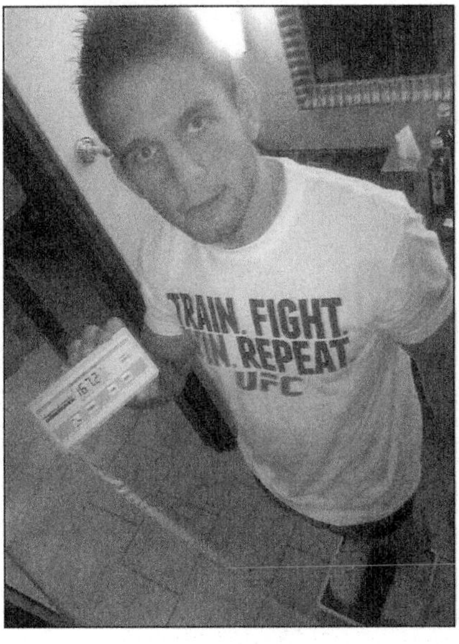

Lentz tips the scale at 167.2 lbs. (right) the same evening after weighing in at 145 lbs. (above)

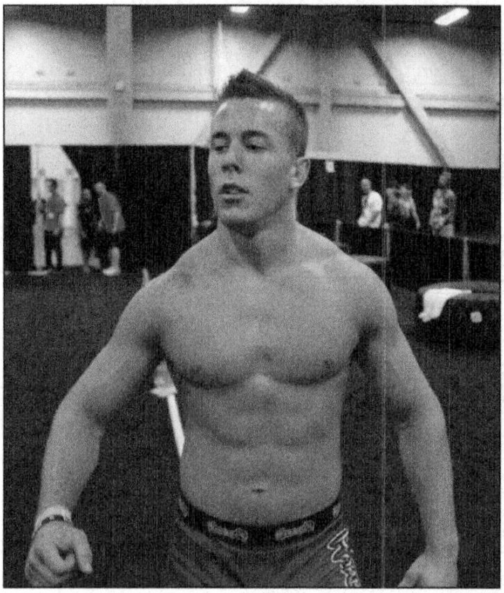

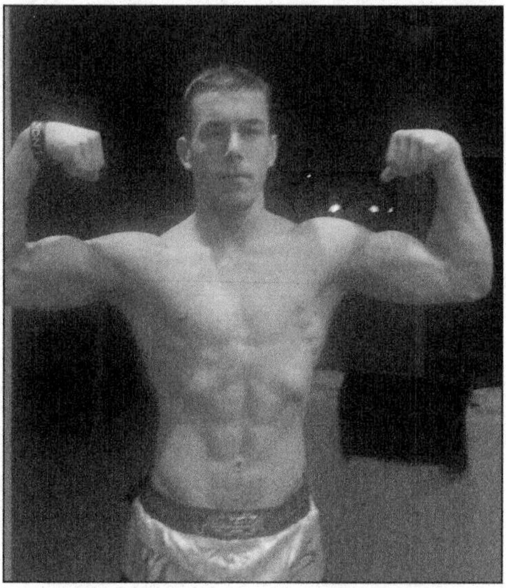

Ridge Kiley used 3 Weeks to Shredded to cut weight for wrestling, shrinking down through multiple weight classes from 165 lbs. to 141 lbs.

RIDGE KILEY

Starting weight: 170 lbs. • Ending weight: 185lbs.

I wrestled at 133 lbs. in 2011 and 2012 for the University of Nebraska. Within 5 months of the 2012 season I was weighing 170 lbs. with only 6.5 percent body fat, and had outgrown multiple weight classes.

Going into my 5th and final year, I desired to compete at 149 lbs. or 157 lbs. but the team was strongest with me at 141 lbs. This is where Mike Dolce came in. I ordered Living Lean and 3 Weeks to Shredded.

Over the course of 1 month I was able to shrink my body from 165 to 141 lbs. while feeling great! During the season, I was able to maintain a healthy range for my weight class, which resulted in a fairly easy weight cut every week.

I am continuing to Live Lean by applying Mike's nutritional principles and will continue to do so the rest of my life.

I wish I had followed these principles earlier in my career because it would have made a huge difference. I underperformed at times because of unhealthy weight-cutting habits. Mike's knowledge could help change the wrestling world!

SLEEP MORE TO LOSE WEIGHT

"Even a soul submerged in sleep is hard at work."
~Heraclitus, 530

As I write, I'm sitting on a plane, flying over the Nevada desert on my way home from an amazing 2-day seminar I conducted for a private group in Southern California. We actually spent quite a bit of time discussing the need for proper sleep. The higher your quality of sleep, the faster your fat loss and muscle growth. Sleep is when our bodies finally have a chance to repair and regenerate from all the hard training.

I function my best with 9 hours of sleep and if you think that makes me lazy, you should see what I accomplish in the 15 hours that I'm awake! In fact, I always had trouble getting rid of that last little bit of belly fat when I was 'only' sleeping 7 hours per night, even though my diet and training was perfect.

As soon as I bumped it up to 9 hours, the fat fell off, the muscle piled on, and I was much more effective in business and at home.

As we age, we tend to sleep less. This means our body is not repairing and regenerating tissue at a rate necessary to outpace aging. It is also not building bones and muscles, and in fact, our strength and skeletal fortitude begin to weaken and become frail. How many 80-year-olds do you see walking around that look like a good breeze could blow them away? That wasn't the case 30 or 40 years ago when they were exiting the prime of their lives.

It is my opinion that time does not age us, our habits do. Habits are very much responsible for our level of health.

I call this your biological age. How old are your cells? How healthy? How vibrant? How efficient?

Think of your cells as a work force at a major manufacturing plant. Each cell is primed and excited, working at a thunderous pace with smiles on their little cell faces as they hum along completing their duties.

Now picture those same workers with beer bellies and cigarettes sticking out of their mouths. How hard do you think they'll be working? How happy will they be? Do you think the quality of their work may suffer?

What happens if some of them stop showing up for work? A few per day, and then soon entire departments, and lastly, the whole plant shuts down.

I prefer to constantly bring in fresh new workers in the way of Earth-grown nutrients, proper rest and big smiles to all those around me.

This is why I always say that The Dolce Diet is not a diet, but a lifestyle. Most people think about losing weight and they only think about food and maybe some form of exercise. Rarely does one think about rest and recuperation.

PAUL HACKETT

Starting weight: 219 lbs. • Ending weight: 171 lbs.

I started by purchasing Living Lean, as I knew it was a winning combination of learning about Mike's journey, motivation, information, and recipes. I then bought the Living Lean Cookbook to get more recipe ideas (as well as incorporating my own ideas whilst maintaining The Dolce Diet principles). I also bought 3 Weeks to Shredded early on, and use it fairly sparingly when needed for fast results.

I have always been a gym rat, whether it was bodybuilding and powerlifting earlier in my life, or my relatively new-found passion of Mixed Martial Arts and sports performance.

I have always "known" the importance of nutrition, but never fully understood the "how" and "why". Because of this, my powerlifting days were where I ate most foods just to get the calories and "nutrients," not too dissimilar to Mike - big and powerful but not exactly a cover model look!

My bodybuilding phase was brief, mainly because the diets I followed were not sustainable and not enjoyable, but also because the workouts were all about aesthetics rather than performance. I felt weaker than during my powerlifting phase, but looked better.

I soon realized that looking good was not enough for me. I don't want bulging biceps and a barrel-chest if it means I am sacrificing performance. We've all seen those dudes in the gym who are HUGE, but lack the flexibility to even take their shirt off after a workout, or not be functionally strong enough to even do a pull up! I did not want to be one of these guys.

I have always had a competitive edge, so I tried my hand at MMA (I had some experience in kickboxing and wrestling, but nothing substantial). I fell in love

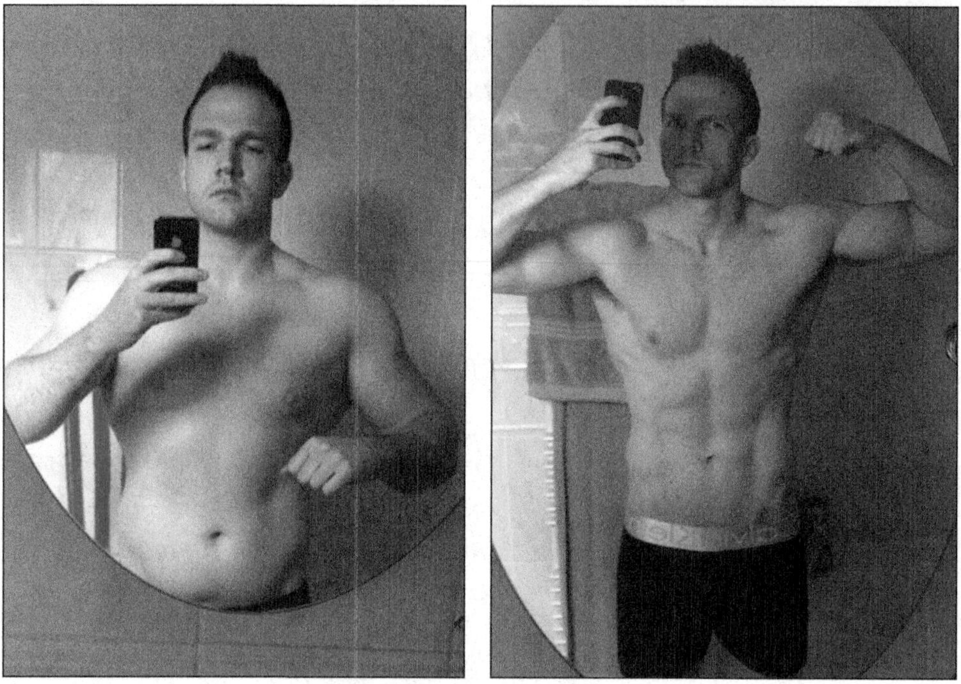

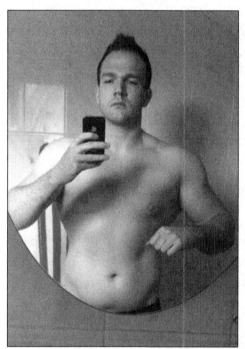

Paul Hackett before The Dolce Diet at 219 lbs. and after at 171 lbs.

with the constant steep learning curve and competitive-but-friendly and respectful nature of all the students I worked with.

But this is where I began to eat more and more again. I wanted to be the biggest and strongest guy in the gym. You might out-strike me, you might outgrapple me, but you will NOT overpower me. So I reverted to a similar mindset to my powerlifting days, which was a mistake.

With my strength (and weight) up, I felt like a monster. Some of the guys at the gym called me "Baby-Brock" in reference to the man-mountain Brock Lesnar. I loved this, but soon grew tired with feeling lethargic throughout the day, particularly after workouts and after eating. By chance, I stumbled across a review online of The Dolce Diet: 3 Weeks to Shredded. I decided to purchase it, along with Living Lean. This is where my performance goals, aesthetic goals, and life goals all aligned and became one newly obtainable goal.

I began using the Living Lean recipes, admittedly finding my favorites and never really trying many new ones, but when it was THIS tasty and produced THESE kind of results, why change?!

In the winter of 2012, I was hovering around the 210-220 lbs. mark. Strong, plenty of lean mass, but covered in a snug blanket of NON-FUNCTIONAL MASS. (This is fat to those who are wondering.) After only a week on the Living Lean lifestyle (it's not a diet!), my energy was through the roof! No lethargy at ANY time of day and no cravings for crappy food. (There were a few in the first few days, but thanks to The Mike Dolce Show podcasts, my eyes were opened to just how awful some foods were; not just the obvious ones like fast food, which I never liked anyway, but foods which seem relatively healthy were suddenly stricken from my vocabulary). I felt like a new man even in the first few weeks.

My training partners began asking what I was doing differently, as my energy was up (both in terms of having a brighter personality and improved cognitive functioning, and also my conditioning), and my body composition was changing rapidly; I was every bit as strong as before, but leaning out and maintaining functional mass. I was soon weighing under 200 lbs., then I was under 190, 180...until I reached what I consider to be my natural weight of around 170-175 lbs. It is at this weight that I feel my strongest and healthiest.

With my training going so well, I decided to do a couple of test weight-cuts to gauge where I would fit in terms of weight classes. I wanted to trial it on my own, without the help of 3 Weeks to Shredded. The idea of weight cutting might sound easy to some (it did to me, to a degree), but MAN is it anything but easy!

With my walk-around weight at about 170, I thought I would get to 155 easy. No dice! I went back to feeling lethargic and lifeless, and on the "deadline day" of my test weight cut, I weighed 158 whilst feeling pretty drawn-out. I was a long way from the UFC, but if I was there, I would likely be cut for being so goddamn unprofessional.

So many people judge fighters for missing weight, and while it is unprofessional (imagine walking in to your office job without your briefcase, or completely naked! UNPROFESSIONAL, right?), it is not obvious to most people watching just how hard a weight cut is.

I dusted myself off, spent the following few weeks building my body back up and repairing the damage I had done over the previous few weeks, then decided to give 3 Weeks to Shredded a go.

Day 1, I woke up and weighed myself. 169 lbs. I followed the information Mike provided in the book (he is not telling you what to eat, he is telling you what worked for him and his athletes). I had energy, just like when following the Living Lean lifestyle; I had strength, just like when following the Living Lean lifestyle; but my body was changing rapidly. I was leaning out and for the first time ever I had abs! Even during my wannabe bodybuilder days, I would struggle to get abs even with the typical "chicken and broccoli" lifestyle. But now I HAVE ABS AND I AM ENJOYING MY FOOD.

I was sure to follow every detail of the 3 Weeks to Shredded guide, as I was certain that Mike's knowledge of nutrients, as well as nutrient timing and manipulation, would make the difference. The third week involved skewing some of the foods to manipulate the way in which my body functioned and reacted with the liquids I was putting into it. The weight was falling off but I still felt ALIVE and STRONG.

WEIGH IN DAY. I woke up, weighed myself, I WAS 153! I WAS BELOW MY TARGET WEIGHT OF 155! I hadn't even resorted to any cardio or sweating processes. I had a quarter cup of black coffee, and headed to the gym to do some light jogging and hill walks, when I was done, I stripped down and weighed myself. 146 lbs. I had just became a featherweight!

Thanks to Living Lean and 3 Weeks to Shredded, I am always avery healthy 170 lbs. guy, with ever-improving strength and performance output, and make 145 lbs. easily and SAFELY.... all while LOOKING GREAT. On top of all of this (yes, there's more!), I feel great. I am happy, confident, bright, and the amount of money I am constantly saving thanks to only buying the affordable foods, but I'm not buying supplements!

I am not the typical dangerously overweight "I need to lose weight to save my life" person, nor am I the supreme athlete who needs the extra kick in the butt. I am like most of you; a fairly healthy human being who didn't realize his full physical and physiological potential until he fed his body the right way, the DOLCE WAY, with real foods.

I tell you this because there may be those of you who don't feel the need to be better, to be healthier. There may be some who wish to give up when they give in to a craving. Some of you may not find the motivation to work out as often as you would like. Whatever your challenge or obstacle, eating Earth-grown nutrients and following Mike Dolce's principles will make you better, make you fitter, make you brighter.

When all of these pieces start falling into place, you will WANT to be better, you will FIND the motivation and time to be more active. No matter your goal, no matter your starting weight or physical condition, these foods will only serve to make you the best you possible. AND WHO DOESN'T WANT THAT? Happy health, everybody.

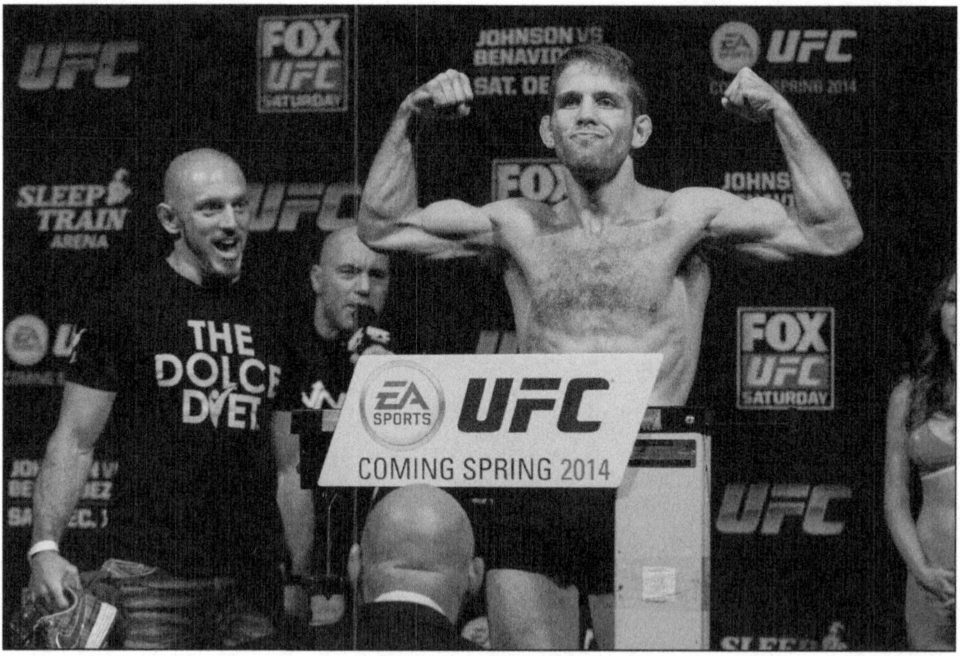

Nik Lentz weighs in for UFC on FOX 9 on Saturday, December 14, 2013.

EATING FOR THE WEIGHT CUT

Weight cutting can and should be an advantage if approached properly. If we only focus on the scale, performance is severely jeopardized, as is often seen at every level of sport. How many times have we heard about a weight cut adversely affecting an athlete's performance?

I look at weight cutting as a chance to purify the system, to detoxify it of any impurities and fill it back up with the highest quality of nutrients at the most crucial time.

The most common dietary practice in the weight-cutting world is to simply drop carbohydrate and water intake in the days and weeks before weigh-ins to reduce bodyweight. If we are only focused on the scale, this method can work, but if we are concerned with maintaining vibrant health and producing a career defining performance, you may want to think twice.

Carbohydrates are turned into glucose and are commonly classified in two categories, complex and simple.

Complex carbohydrates are often found in:
Grains: oats, quinoa, rice
Beans: black, pinto, garbanzo
Vegetables: potatoes, peas, corn

Simple carbohydrates are often found in fruits such as blueberries and strawberries or even raw honey.

Complex carbohydrates are not readily available and must be broken down in the digestive system before they can be utilized as energy. Simple carbohydrates offer a more immediate energy supply.

What do carbohydrates do in the body? For starters, they are stored in

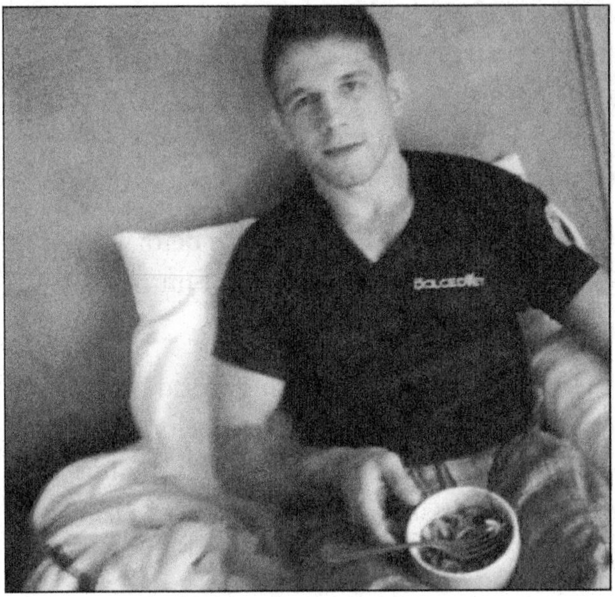

Nik "The Carny" Lentz enjoys a signature Dolce Diet Breakfast Bowl the day before weigh-ins.

muscles as glycogen for sustained contractions. Pretty important for athletes, don't you think?

Next, they are used by your organs to facilitate proper function and sustained health.

Last, and most important, glucose is the primary fuel source for the brain. The brain, of course, is central command, headquarters, and the control room. If the power goes out in the control room, the brain will start shutting down areas of the body it deems less important than itself - and the brain indeed deems EVERY other part of the body less important. Based upon the limited fuel the brain has available, it may start shutting off areas of the body that are pretty darn necessary, like the heart, kidneys, muscles, lungs, vision or many other debilitating areas. How many zombies have you seen getting ready for bodybuilding competitions? Or what about the girl at work making a dozen errors per day while she's trying to shrink down for vacation?

In MMA, you see these mindless zombies walking into walls during fight week as they hunt down a Starbucks hoping the coffee will act like jumper cables on their brain.

In my experience, carbohydrate intake should be based upon energy expenditure. We do not indiscriminately limit our carbs; we eat based upon our need. (Dolce Diet Principle #2!)

For example, my athletes will often share videos or Tweets during fight week showing their meals such as pancakes, oatmeal bowls, pasta dishes and tons of fruit only to be inundated with questions as to how this is possible?!

"Don't you have a fight coming up?"

The answer is YES, and that is exactly WHY we are eating like this. I know it is a different activity, but the same principle holds true for endurance athletes increasing their carbohydrate content prior to competition. They do so in an attempt to pack their energy stores enough to sustain them during their race. Combat athletes are exactly the same, except we step on a scale 24 hours before competition.

ZAC SHEPARD

Starting weight: 195 lbs. • Ending weight: 172 lbs.

After struggling to make weight for my pro debut and being frustrated all the time from being hungry and feeling drained, I was looking into diets that fighters were following to make weight.

After hearing about how much weight Thiago Alves and Johny Hendricks were cutting, seeing how heavy they were going into their fight, and noticing how well they were performing, I looked into the Dolce Diet. Coincidently, one of my brothers already had Mike's books. I came across 3 Weeks to Shredded, gave it a try, and never looked back.

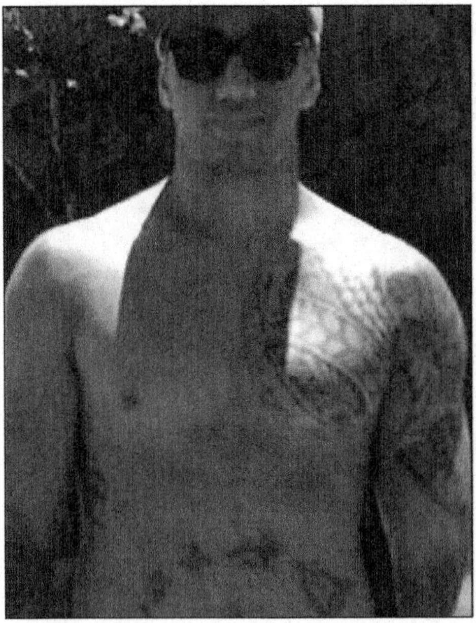

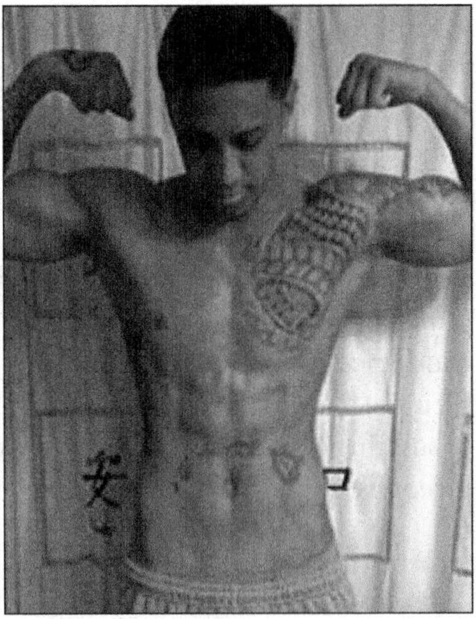

Zac Shepard before The Dolce Diet at 195 lbs. and after at 172 lbs.

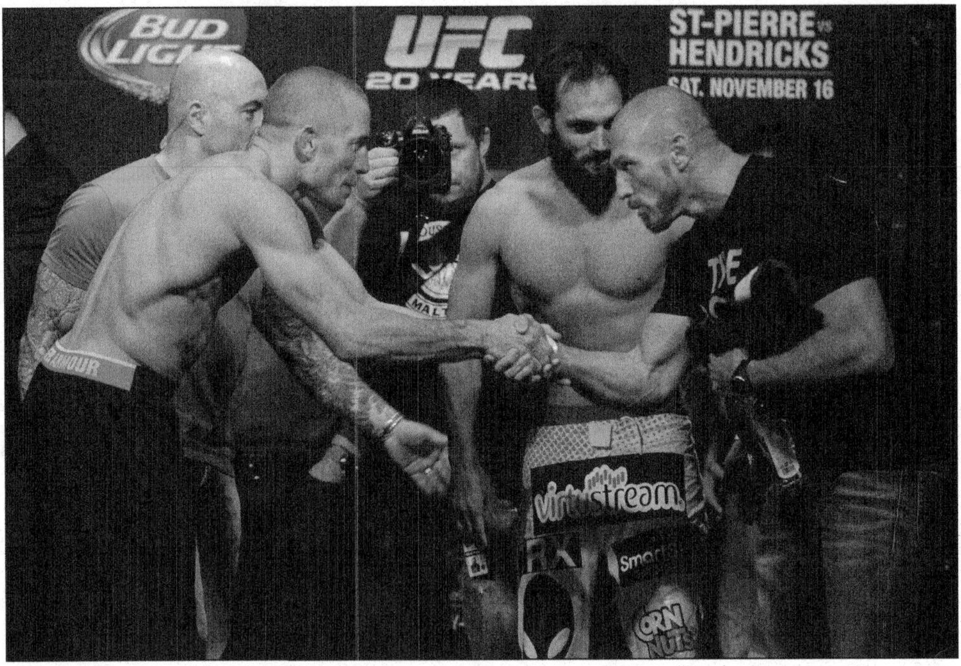

Georges St. Pierre vs. Johny Hendricks took place November 16, 2013.

THE WEIGHT CUT & WATER

> *"We forget that the water cycle and the life cycle are one."*
> *~Jacques Cousteau*

Water must be consumed at all times. But why, Mike? <insert whiney voice here> Why do I have to drink so much water? I hear it ALL THE TIME!

Well, you don't have to. You don't HAVE to do anything. But here is why we should: Water will cleanse your entire body from the inside out. It will provide satiation to your hunger, improve cardio-respiratory function and facilitate a healthy skeletal system.

When I begin the weight-cut process, I will kick my personal water intake up to 20 lbs. per day (over 2.5 gallons). My athletes do the same. Now, the athletes I work with typically train 3 times per day and utilize the hot tub and cold baths to recuperate, but my point is to drink much more water than you currently are.

I always have "lbs." of water everywhere I go. My kitchen, my office, my cars, my gym bag, my backpack, my locker and in my hand! I find it best to purchase my water in cases of 16 oz. bottles. I also carry a 40 oz. stainless steel canteen in my backpack and fill it every chance I get. I take full responsibility for my hydration and ensure I'm never without a clean, refreshing drink.

As long as you are urinating properly, it is extremely hard to drink too much water. When it comes to the weight cut, it is a pretty simple concept that if you eliminate consumption and continue expenditure, you will deplete supplies. This practice is also used adversely to prepare for competition. Athletes simply stop drinking water a few days (sometimes weeks) before competition to deplete their body of water and thus achieve a lighter weight. What they fail to realize is that water is essential for nearly every cellular function. The human body, by the way, is nothing more than a compilation of cells.

By reducing water, you are also reducing the ability of your body to perform. Do you see where I'm going with this? By reducing carbohydrates and water, the body is less able to perform in a healthy manner, leading to a torturous weight cut and incomplete rehydration.

To me, it always made the most sense to keep the athlete fed during the final few days, so he would have the strength and the mental acuity to perform the task at hand. By keeping the athlete extremely hydrated, the body would not react adversely when we temporarily purge it of water. In fact, the body will give it freely.

It is not uncommon for my athletes to drink 2 to 3 gallons of water per day up until the night before weigh-ins. Have you noticed how many trips to the bathroom you make when you are drinking in excess of 2 gallons per day?! A good rule of thumb is to always be urinating clearly, with the exception of your morning trip to the bathroom.

Now, how do we pull the water off?

There are a few ways that some athletes prefer. I have my own personal favorite, but I allow for the confidence of the athlete. Some athletes like to train at low intensity in hot rooms with sweatpants on. This certainly works, but is often too taxing. Other athletes prefer to walk on a treadmill in plastic suits. This is also effective, but if you have more than 5 lbs. to lose, you could be in for a long day.

Some use the old approach of sitting in a sauna, which I least prefer. A sauna should be for relaxing. You might as well rub butter all over yourself and jump into the oven because you are cooking yourself. There are more missed weights and panic attacks from the sauna than any other routine I know about, and I always try to talk anyone out of going this route.

A more preferred method is using a spa or hot tub. This is a rather gentle way to break and maintain a sweat while breathing comfortable, room temperature air and simply being able to step out and jump into the pool to cool off.

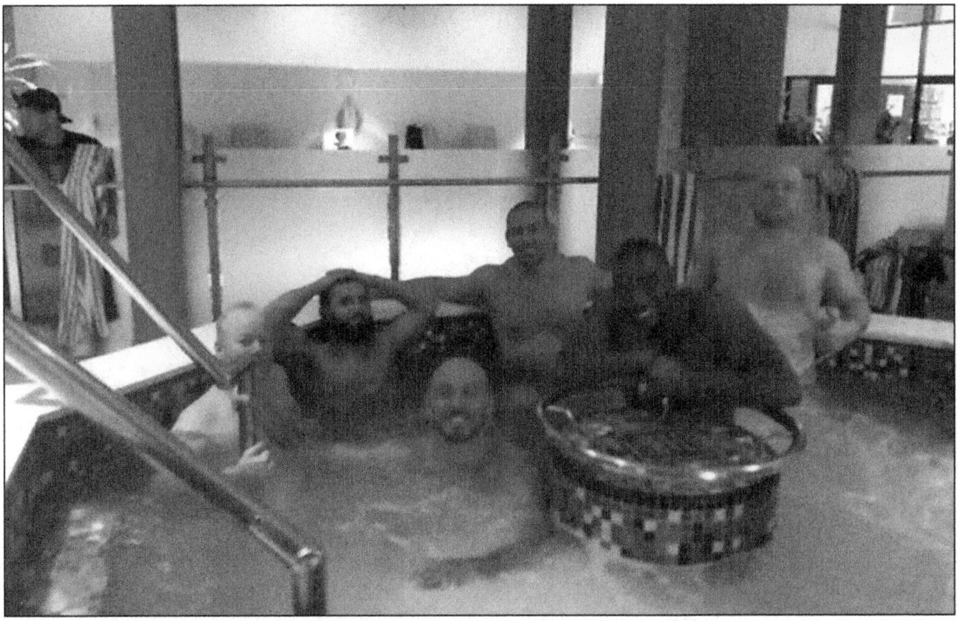

Coach Mike Dolce, Johny "Bigg Rigg" Hendricks and Team Takedown sit in the hot tub to cut weight. The team uses this time to bond and support their teammate.

THE DOLCE STEP METHOD

Weight cutting is a very lonely process, often torturous. I try to alleviate the stress, anxiety and discomfort of my athletes by continuously seeking new ways to lose weight while increasing comfort and confidence. My preferred method we call The Dolce Step Method. Locking an athlete in a sauna while the teams and coaches sit outside the door will never be seen in a Dolce weight cut. What will be seen is the athlete, myself and usually each member of the team hanging out in the pool area laughing, listening to music and losing weight…without even knowing it. The following method I found to be the easiest and most natural way of losing weight while keeping the athlete surrounded by those who care most about his health and well-being.

The Dolce Step Method

Step 1
Get in a hot tub and submerge yourself to your neck for 5 minutes.

Step 2
Next, sit on the bottom stair so the water is at chest level for another 5 minutes.

Step 3
Then, move up one stair so the water is now at belly button level.

Step 4
Next, move up another stair to where just your glutes and hamstrings are submerged.

Step 5
Sit outside of the spa with just your feet and calves in.
You have just performed a 25-minute session and continued sweating while not overheating or inducing a state of anxiety.

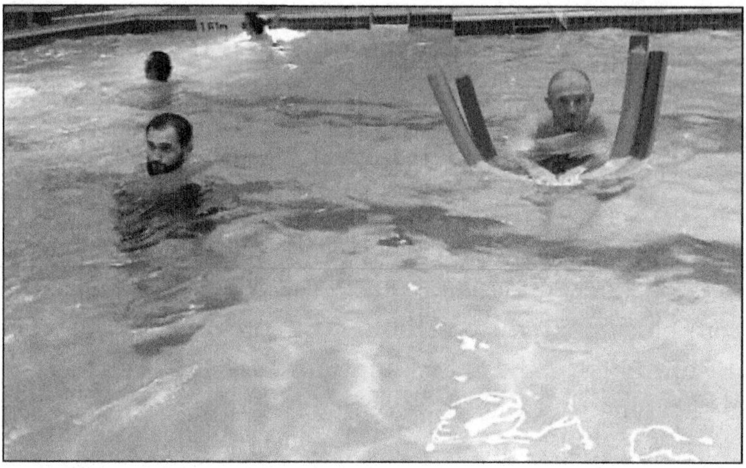

Coach Mike Dolce and Johny Hendricks finish a weight-cut session with a cool dip in the pool.

Step 6
For the last 5 minutes, jump into a cold pool and cool yourself down completely. This is usually good for shedding 2-4 lbs. in 30 minutes. That is a 3 lbs. average.

Repeat twice and you have just cut 6 lbs. in an hour.

That is about the limit of what I would like to cut on weigh-in day.

If you are in really bad shape, this method can easily pull upwards of 10 lbs. off in 2 hours or so. However, it is my intention to only lose 2 to 4 lbs. on weigh-in day.

Thiago Alves woke up "on weight" for the UFC Fox 11 card, and not many athletes are as big as Thiago relative to their weight class.

THE DOLCE STEP METHOD

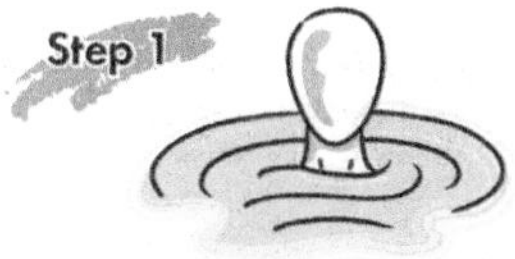

Get in a hot tub and submerge yourself to your neck for 5 minutes.

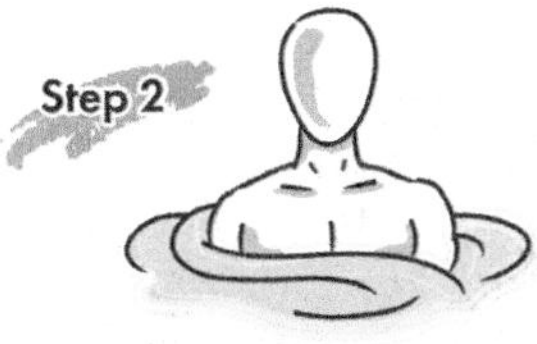

Next, sit on the bottom stair so the water is at chest level for another 5 minutes.

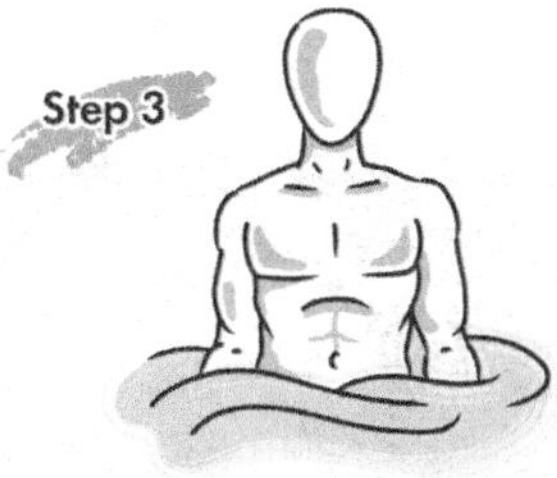

Then, move up one stair so the water is now at belly button level.

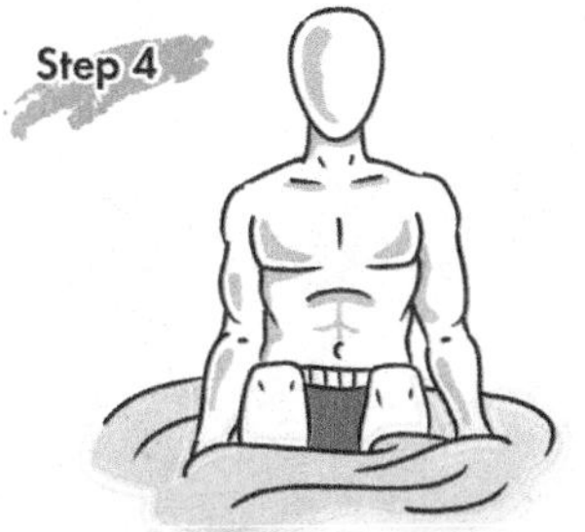

Next, move up another stair to where just your glutes and hamstrings are submerged.

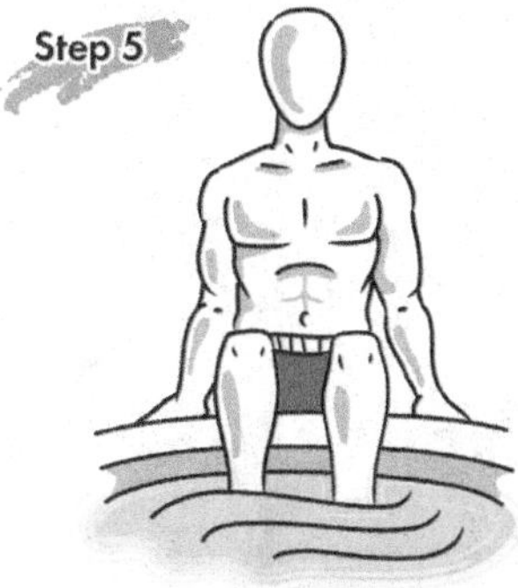

Last, sit outside of the spa with just your feet and calves in.

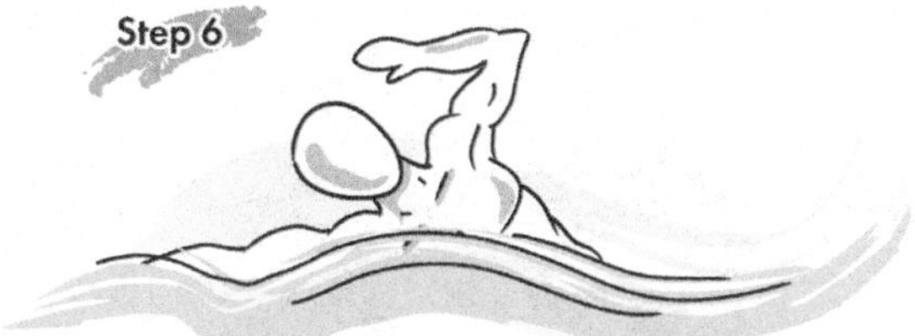

For the last 5 minutes, jump into a cold pool and cool yourself down completely. This is usually good for shedding 2-4 lbs. in 30 minutes. That is a 3 lbs. average.

You have just performed a 25-minute session and continued sweating while not overheating or inducing a state of anxiety.

JAMIE KIENHOLZ

Starting weight: 130 lbs. • Ending weight: 125 lbs.

I doubled up 3 Weeks to Shredded (6 weeks) to drop weight for my first bikini competition. I was able to continue to train hard and maintained my energy level throughout my cutting.

The process worked so well, that I was actually too muscular for my category, and now I will be moving up to compete at the figure level.

Thanks, Dolce!

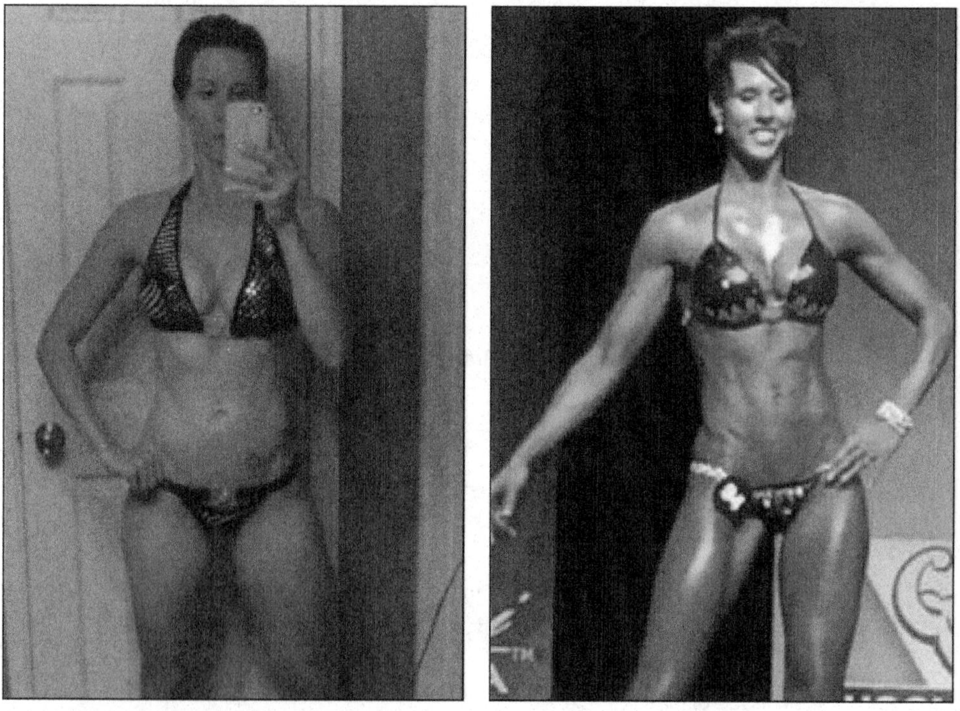

Jamie Kienholz before The Dolce Diet at 130 lbs. and after at 125 lbs.

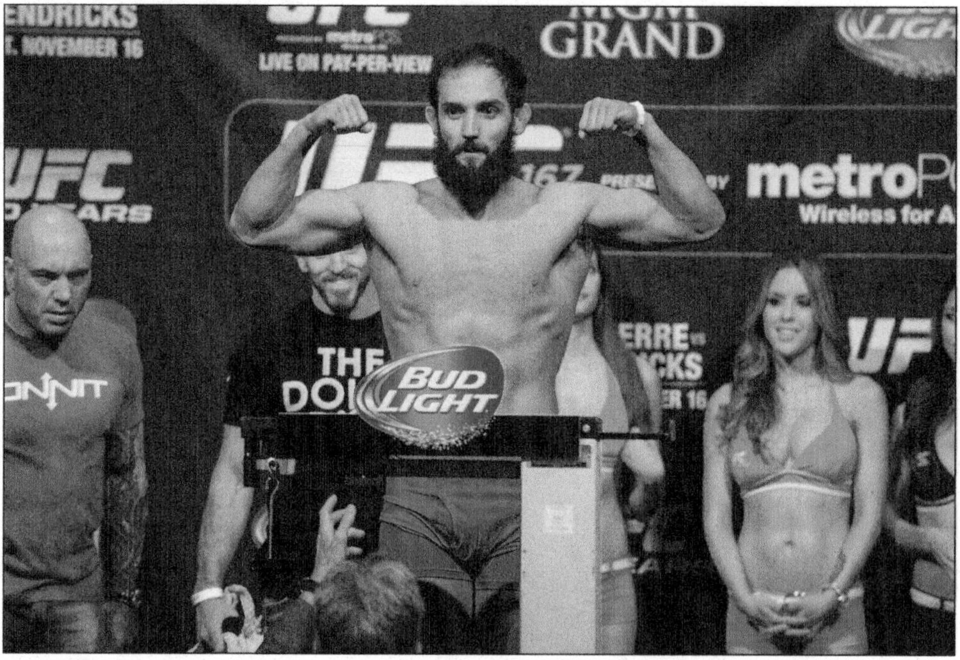

Johny "Bigg Rigg" Hendricks completes another successful weigh-in.

REHYDRATION: WHAT TO EAT & DRINK AFTER STEPPING OFF THE SCALE

UFC weigh-ins are really something to experience, especially from behind the curtain. The number of folks who will actually experience that is few. Picture 30 or so wrung-out guys, standing with their plus-one or coach. Their name is called. The curtain opens. They walk out. Those at home hear the roar of the crowd, Joe Rogan's introduction and announcement of weight. But in a bad weight cut, the fighter hears none of that; maybe a ringing, maybe some muffled undertones. It's difficult to tell what a fighter is feeling when he steps onto that scale, but most of the time, it's not good. However, when a weight cut is done properly, you can tell. The confidence is written all over the athlete's face. In this chapter, I want to discuss what a successful rehydration should mean to you.

All too often, I have seen elite athletes, Pay-Per-View superstars, step off the scale, walk behind the curtain and immediately grab a box of take-out pasta from the nearest restaurant and devour it with a popular, chemically flavored 'sport rehydration' drink.

Not long after, I see the same athlete lying on the floor, legs up in the air and in obvious digestive discomfort, as their body tries to understand why the heck its master has tried to poison it. Soon after, this same athlete will often be found making one of many trips to the restroom to dispose of these poisons in one of two ways. Both are undesirable!

Remember, it is not what we consume, but what we absorb, that matters! I want my athletes to always be a little hungry and keep the food moving through their systems as they get closer to weigh-in day. Post weigh-in, the key to healthy rehydration is to back out of the weight cut the same way you pulled in. This means sticking with the same foods you've been eating all week, and further, all training camp. That way, there are no surprises, and the body is able to efficiently absorb these known nutrients.

You might be surprised at the number of world-class athletes pulling out bags of food from the local hotel deli and eating white bread turkey sandwiches with mayonnaise and french fries, or fettuccine Alfredo and spaghetti and meatballs from the local pasta shop. Unfortunately, I love it, because I know it's not my guy. The reason we conduct the weight cut the way we do is to create an advantage for my athlete.

I will work 10,000 hours to gain 1 second of advantage because a split second can win a world title. That is the philosophy we bring into the weight cut. We don't cut corners. We don't hope for "good enough." We only do what is best. When an athlete steps off the scale, they've only 50 percent completed their contracted task. Now they must rehydrate as perfectly as they trained in order to perform at their peak levels.

Treat the rehydration process with the same reverence and discipline as you would every other aspect of your training. Far too many fights have been lost in the 24 hours after weigh-ins than in the 15 minutes contested in the ring. Off the scale, it is time to begin hydrating. The human body needs oxygen, water and food in that order to survive and thrive. Rehydrating is no different. The oxygen should be pretty simple. The water should be, too. Begin sipping slowly. It's much better to take 1 sip every minute than to finish an entire glass in a gulp. Too much fluid too soon - especially if there are nerves in the air - can cause an upset stomach very quickly. The digestive system relies on proper blood volume in order to adequately process the food you'll be consuming. Oftentimes when cutting weight, an athlete may be dehydrated, which can result in an unfavorable blood volume. This state can adversely affect efficient digestion. Therefore, we begin rehydrating slowly.

My athletes are reminded to eat in handfuls of our approved food list every 5 to 15 minutes, as they feel necessary. There is no hard and fast rule here as one athlete may only be losing 8 lbs. while another may be losing 28 lbs. Eating in handfuls allows a simple unit of measure and keeps the athlete consistently refueling while not overeating or slowing (or even halting) the digestive process.

Most often, when an athlete steps off the scale, he is in a mild state of dehydration. The body needs to establish a favorable balance of water before our systems will begin functioning normally, especially when it comes to the digestive system. As any survivalist knows, a human being can

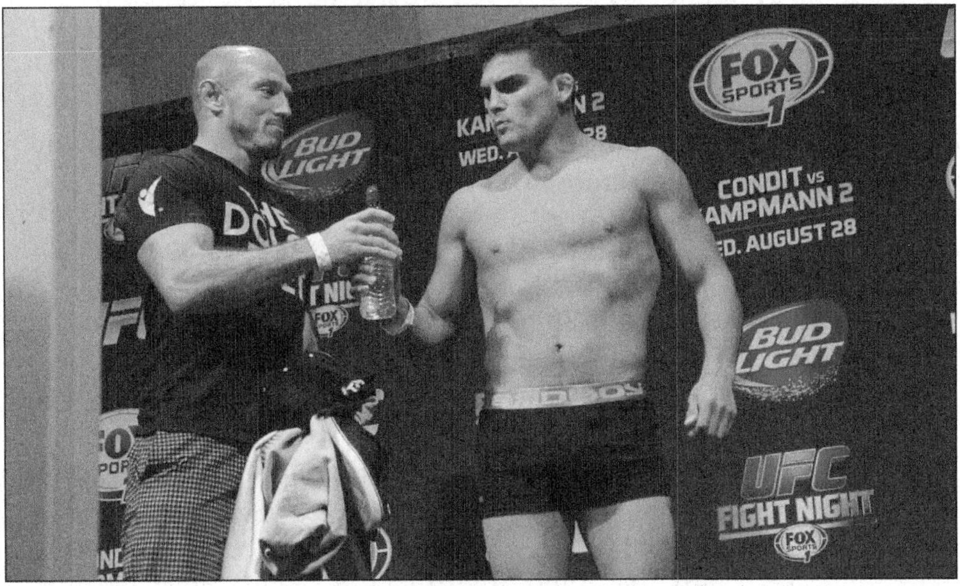

Welterweight Kelvin Gastelum takes a sip of Mike Dolce's Electrolyte Drink after stepping off the scale. Gastelum won The Ultimate Fighter Season 17 as a middleweight and then dropped a weight class to 170 lbs. He currently is undefeated.

live for weeks on little-to-no calories. But, take the water away, and we are dead within a few days. This is a universal concept we should always consider.

Our emotional side is what craves the food, but if an athlete walked into a hospital in the same dehydrated state, the doctors would immediately act to replenish the fluids and electrolytes and not hand them a plate of pasta. When my athletes step off the stage, we immediately begin to rehydrate with (go ahead, take a guess) WATER!

I've discussed how important it is for athletes to be eating during their weight cuts to ensure they are healthy and strong. You should be hungry on weigh-in day but not starving. If you are starving at the scale, you probably starved yourself to get there.

Having established the hierarchy of fluids over food in an elite rehydration program, we must discuss the types of fluids. This is where I will stand up on my soap box and preach until you are sick of hearing me talk.

I am a longevity advocate, an advocate of Earth-grown nutrients and an advocate of lifelong health.

As such, I cannot suggest you reach for a manmade concoction of chemicals, colorings and contaminants over the tried and true combination of H2O, which has sustained all of life on this planet since the dawn of time. Let me say that again…Water has sustained all of life on this planet since the dawn of time!

Why would we believe that some guy with a few patents, an advertising department, a graphic designer, scores of focus groups and the self-serving interest of financial profits, has created a product that is better than plain old, freely available, "untrademarkable" water!?

Do you get my point? Water is the key to life and the key to a successful rehydration. Off the scale, drink slowly but consistently. Now it is time to introduce familiar foods into your digestive system. I say familiar foods because we must only consume foods that have been regularly processed by our digestive systems so there are no malfunctions. Again, we want to stick as close as possible to our standard ingredient list we used during our training camp.

As a general rule, we should begin with simple sugars to peak energy levels and turn on the metabolism, while being easy for the body to break down and absorb. A great choice might be orange slices, applesauce, berries or melon. Next we can move to more complex carbs like brown rice, quinoa, oat bran or sweet potatoes.

Finally, when a good portion of our weight has come back on and we are feeling ourselves again, you can test a small portion of a regular meal. Something you would eat any night of your last hard training week. For my athletes, we usually enjoy my Power Pasta recipe (The Dolce Diet: Living Lean Cookbook), which is packed with all the essential nutrients you will need to fully replenish your nutrient stores and is absolutely delicious!

NOTE: See the recipe for Mike Dolce's Natural Electrolyte Drink in Part 3

"As I see it, every day you do one of two things: build health or produce disease in yourself." ~Adelle Davis

Part II

THE ORIGINAL
3 WEEKS TO SHREDDED PROGRAM

THE ORIGINAL 3 WEEKS TO SHREDDED PROGRAM

This is the original version of the 3 Weeks to Shredded program written in 2007. This program is still extremely effective and has been used by hundreds of thousands of people around the world, making it an international bestseller. Consider the principles and techniques used as valuable tools for your next weight cut.

Let's Get Going

You and I are starting a journey together. You know your goals. Now how are you going to achieve them? To get to where we're going, we have to know what it is that's standing between us and our destination.

Open your cabinets and pantry. Take everything out and put it on the counters and table.

Now, open up your refrigerator and do the same. Everything comes out.

Take a good look at everything. This is what your organs, your bones, your muscles, your dreams and your realities are all made of. Everything we put into our bodies becomes absorbed by our bodies, regardless of its ability to make us healthy or sick, stronger or weaker.

We are what we eat in a very literal sense. Everything we ingest changes us.

Do you feel fresh and vibrant or old and tired? How about right now, at this very moment? Close your eyes and hold a firm picture of how you look in your mind, and now look again at everything you removed from your cabinets and refrigerator.

Locate any products that you feel may be holding you back from reaching your goals? And be generous with your accusations. You're right.

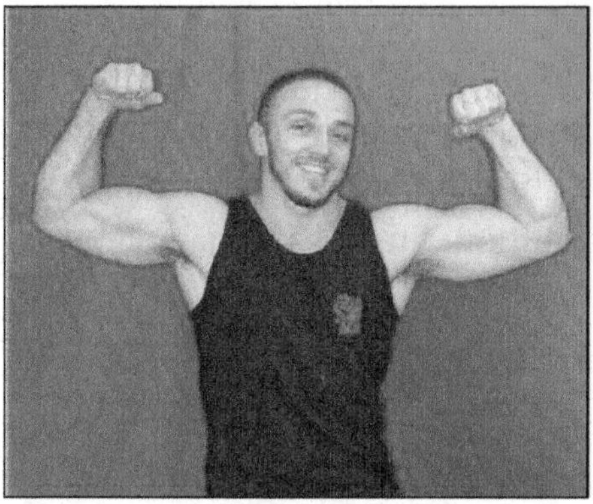

Mike Dolce at 220 lbs. Mike began his original 3 Weeks to Shredded weight cut at 212.8 lbs.

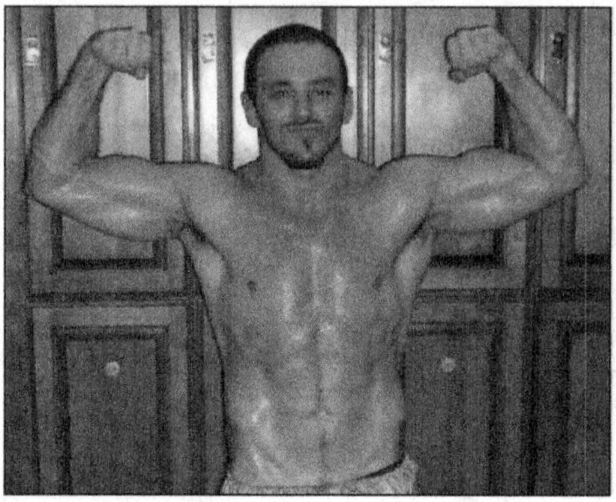

Mike at 185 lbs.

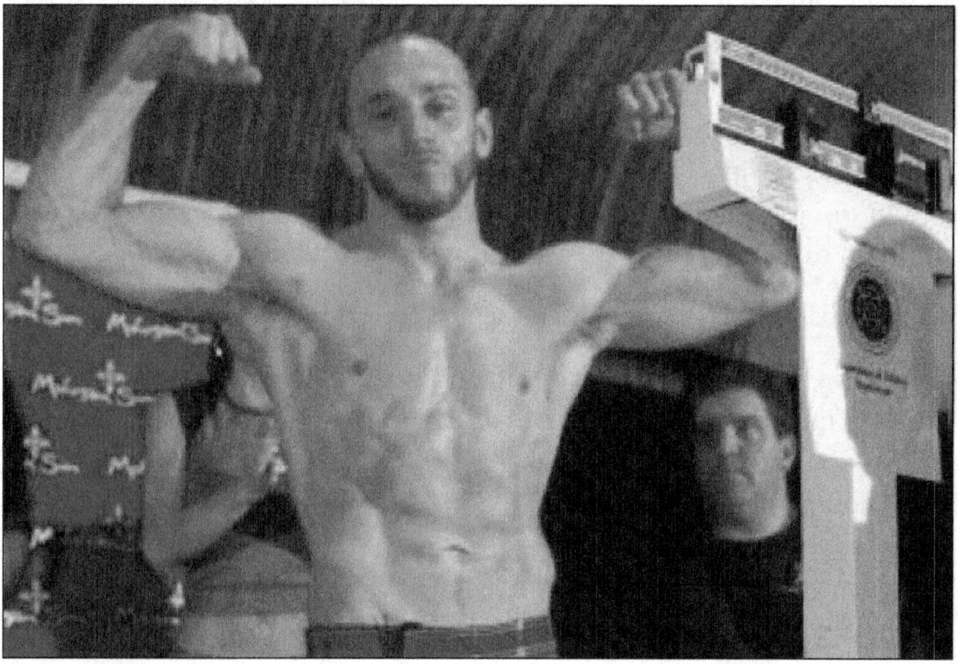

Mike at 170 lbs.

Any cookies, cakes, tarts, treats, chocolate, candy, pretzels, popcorn, chips, bread, creams, jellies, ice cream, crackers, butter, margarine, cooking oils or anything else that would fit nicely into this group?

If so, THROW IT OUT, RIGHT NOW! That's right, put it all in the garbage, where it belongs. We're going to rebuild your life together, and never look back!

Now take a look at what's left. With the garbage out of the way, let's identify the products that may improve your chances of reaching your goals. What do you think?

Fresh foods like vegetables, fruits, legumes, nuts, seeds, eggs, fish, and grass-fed meats should be at the top of that list, though we respond differently to specific items and should choose accordingly.

As a rule, we should always consume the freshest, most natural, and least treated items available to us…Earth-grown nutrients!

If it wasn't available 200 years ago, you shouldn't be eating it today. Typically, the more a food product is handled, the lower its nutrient value will be. Knowing that, we can determine that the closer a food product is to its most natural form and habitat, the greater the nutritional value.

These "common sense" tips will prove invaluable as you begin to determine your own nutritional style. My personal diet consists of about 80 percent organic ingredients, but as a rule, I will only eat fresh, 100 percent organic fruits and vegetables. I always buy local and prefer the least invasive forms of preparation.

Now, put everything back where it belongs. Have you noticed that your cabinets are looking a bit bare? So will your waistline!

GET ON BOARD!

If you live with friends or family members, please pay close attention to the following advice. Call a house meeting. It won't take more than 20 seconds or so. Gather all of your housemates together and tell them that you have set a very important goal for yourself.

You can tell them what your goal is or you can simply say that you've set a personal goal, and you need their help. They don't have to eat what you do, but they can't share what they are eating with you.

Ask them personally to understand and be supportive of your hard work and please keep all difficult nutritional situations away from you for the next few weeks.

Look them in the eyes and be sincere.

Real friends will be elated and some may even join in as your actions will serve to motivate many, but do not push your lifestyle on anyone.

No matter how well intended, many will resent empathy. Simply go about your day and live by example. Those who will...WILL.

BREAKFAST

Certainly the most important meal of the day is breakfast. If we could only eat a well balanced breakfast, as opposed to a well balanced dinner each day, the breakfast eaters would be much healthier, capable individuals. Trust me. I've tried it.

> ***"It surprises me when a modern adult admits to regularly missing breakfast because of time constraints! How can anyone not have time for breakfast?"***

It surprises me when a modern adult admits to regularly missing breakfast because of time constraints! How can anyone not have time for breakfast? Typically, breakfast is the first meal of the day, hence the first thing you do in a day. You may have places to be after breakfast, but most don't have anywhere to be before breakfast.

Have they tried going to bed 20 minutes earlier each night and waking up 20 minutes earlier each morning? Heck, make it 30 minutes or an hour. Wouldn't the extra quiet time be well worth it?

Most of the world is a big fan of eggs. I am, too. I love omelets, scrambles and wraps. Especially when married to a host of nutritious, fresh vegetables, olives and beans.

Fresh fruit is awesome also! Vibrant colors and anything in season will always fill my morning table.

Water is usually bypassed in the wee hours of the morning unless of course, you are expelling it. Most of the time though, people will go to the coffees, teas and juices before addressing the most basic human need...hydration.

If you are thirsty, you are dehydrated. The first thing you should do each and every morning is drink 16 oz. of room temperature, filtered water. This will clean your digestive tract, begin revitalizing your cells and turn on your metabolism.

Next, prepare your ingredients, turn on the tea pot and take a minute to enjoy the beginning of a wonderful day!

LUNCH

In this day and age, it is very common for us to consider lunch the meal we eat between the hours of 11am and 2pm. I will go along with that, but I do not consider lunch a meal dictated by the nearest fast food restaurant to your office building. Lunch is simply called lunch for the sake of your lunch break.

On The Dolce Diet, lunch will be a very clean, nutritious, simple preparation that you prepare at home and bring with you. It will be very tasty and perfectly proportioned to your needs. Now, it is possible that you can purchase an excellent replica of any number of my meal suggestions in a select few specialty shops, but as a rule, bring your own lunch anyway. Otherwise, you may be forced into a tempting situation.

SNACKS

Snacks are fun! Snacks should always taste good! Snacks have to be nutritious and must be planned. Otherwise, you're grabbing whatever is around, just to hold me over until I get home, or just as bad, you go too long before providing nourishing fuel for yourself, causing a cascade of cellular distress and disease.

And, all of this because you didn't take an extra 32 seconds this morning to throw a handful of raw almonds into a Ziploc bag with a handful of dried cranberries.

We eat snacks as blood sugar stabilizers between our more nutrient-packed meals. Snacks stabilize our metabolism and provide clean energy to our working body. At times, students of mine have tried to skip their snacks, thinking the calorie reduction will speed up weight loss, but in fact, found the opposite to be true. The more often we stoke our metabolism, the hotter it will burn.

DINNER

Dinner serves a similar purpose to lunch and is typically eaten at home with loved ones. Considering you will be breaking bread at this time with those you care most about, don't you want to influence them to be as healthy and fit as possible?

It drives me crazy that most American families are too busy to eat well. Ronald McDonald and Carl's Jr. have taken over the dinner tables of hard working, well intentioned families, and we are dying as a result.

Stop this now! Dinner should be the same size and variety as your lunch. My dinner is very much the same as my lunch, with some creative twists that my palate will enjoy.

Open a recipe book, turn on the computer and type "salad recipe" into your favorite search engine and get cooking. This meal will give you the nutrients you need to rebuild your strength from a long day and revitalize your energy for the day ahead.

*"My body is like breakfast, lunch and dinner.
I don't think about it, I just have it."* -Arnold Schwarzenegger

3 DAYS OF EATING

This is a fun exercise I like to do with my clients.

Write down everything you ate yesterday, today and tomorrow. Include the time of each meal and the exact name and quantity of each item. This will help you understand your habits and troubleshoot your current diet.

Mine might look like this:

3/16/2007

7:15am: 24oz water, 1cup green tea, 5 egg whites, 1/4 red pepper, 1/4 green pepper, 1/4 onion, 1/4 tomato, 1 handful spinach, 1oz feta cheese, 2 whole grain wraps, 1 tbsp extra virgin olive oil

10:30am: 24oz water, 1 cup green tea, 3/4 cup oatmeal, 1 1/2 cup mixed berries, 1 pinch cinnamon

1pm: 24oz water, 1 cup green tea, 2 handfuls field greens, 1/4 red pepper, 1/4 green pepper, 1/4 onion, 1/4 tomato, 1/2 cup chopped broccoli, 3oz black olives, 2 tbsp extra virgin olive oil, 2 tbsp apple cider vinegar, 1/2 cup dried cranberries, 1 handful crushed almonds, 1 tbsp sesame seeds

4pm: 24oz water, 1 cup green tea, 1 slice organic whole grain flax enriched toast, 2 tbsp almond butter, 1/2 cup applesauce

7pm: 24oz water, 6oz dry organic whole grain spaghetti, 1/2 can organic tomato sauce, 1/2 chopped tomato, 1 garlic clove, 1/4 red pepper, 1/4 green pepper, 1/4 onion, 1/2 eggplant, 1 handful field greens, 1tbsp extra virgin olive oil, oregano, basil

10pm: 1/2 cup dry Kashi Autumn Wheat cereal, 1 cup mixed berries, 1 cup 2 percent or less milk

Now it's your turn. Grab a pen and a piece of paper and write down what you ate yesterday and what you've eaten, so far, today. Remember to include the times you ate. This might be difficult for some people because very few people are on an eating schedule. (And you will be soon!) Try your best for now. Be sure to include every single crumb and every beverage! No one will see this but you, so be honest. Put the paper where you will remember it, and tomorrow as you eat, write everything down.

Come back to this section once it's complete.

How do the days differ?

Did you eat the same foods on the third day as you did on the first? Did you not eat breakfast? Maybe you didn't eat all day only to binge eat at 11pm before falling into bed.

Perhaps you ate great! Good for you! Often, seeing what we eat is shocking! Most people tend to forget everything they consume, as well as the amounts.

Paying just a little bit more attention to what we eat can go a long way to managing our weight. If you can't control what you put in your mouth, you can't control anything.

"Habits change into character." ~Ovid

3 DAYS OF EATING

YESTERDAY (Day 1) ____/____/____

____/____/____ ____

____

____/____/____ ____

____

____/____/____ ____

____

____/____/____ ____

____

____/____/____ ____

____

____/____/____ ____

____

____/____/____ ____

____

3 DAYS OF EATING

TODAY (Day 2) ____/____/____

____/____/____ ____

____

____/____/____ ____

____

____/____/____ ____

____

____/____/____ ____

____

____/____/____ ____

____

____/____/____ ____

____

____/____/____ ____

____

3 DAYS OF EATING

TOMORROW (Day 3) ____/____/____

____/____/____ ____

____

____/____/____ ____

____

____/____/____ ____

____

____/____/____ ____

____

____/____/____ ____

____

____/____/____ ____

____

____/____/____ ____

____

EXERCISE

This topic alone is worthy of thousands of books, and I could not do it justice here. Instead, I will offer you the following thoughts and defer to your own resourcefulness to get the job done.

Obviously exercise is important. Everybody knows that. The question lies in the type, frequency, volume and intensity of exercise, for you. Again, what are your goals?

One of my students is 83 years old and has all the typical health concerns. She exercises 4 days per week, water-aerobics, mall walking, horse shoes, and chair Pilates...sometimes more.

Another of my students is 42 and wants to lose 100 lbs. He parks in the lot across the street from his office, instead of at the back door, and walks his dog around his neighborhood (2 miles) 3 times per week...for now.

Most of my athletes train up to 30 hours per week, and they always train hard. Nutrition is most important, but exercise is still in the same sentence.

Everyone should be doing some form of exercise from evening walks to Plyometrics, 3 to 20 exercise sessions per week.

You must be following your personal exercise lifestyle program in order to fully achieve your health goals.

But, you already knew that. Now commit to it.

"A pessimist sees the difficulty in every opportunity; an optimist sees the opportunity in every difficulty." ~ Winston Churchill

3 WEEKS TO SHREDDED MEAL PLAN

In 2007, I was offered a big opportunity on a grand stage in the now defunct International Fight League. Could I fight at welterweight in 6 weeks? At the time that question was asked of me, I was over the class weight limit by more than 40 lbs. but I wasn't going to turn down what I saw as the chance of a lifetime.

So between April 16, 2007 and June 1, 2007 I reduced my bodyweight from 212.8 lbs. to 170 lbs. One day later, on June 2, I competed as a professional mixed martial artist weighing 198 lbs. During the 6 weeks of preparation for this fight and subsequent weigh-in, I had to lose 42.8 lbs. I came down from a very healthy 212.8 lbs. to the welterweight class limit of 170 lbs.

I am a professional and was under strict medical supervision.

My weight loss is neither typical nor expected with this, or any type of program. This information is a retelling of my personal story.

The meals that follow are what I ate everyday, without substitution and without excuse, during the dates indicated.

"The highest levels of performance come to people who are centered, intuitive, creative, and reflective - people who know to see a problem as an opportunity." -Deepak Chopra

WEEK 1 • STARTING THE FIRE

Current weight 197.8 lbs. / 27.8 lbs. to go

My weight might seem high but I feel great and see my body changing everyday. This amount of food keeps me satisfied and energized. The hard part is on the way!

May 10 - 16, 2007
This is the exact meal plan I followed 3 weeks before my weigh-in at 170 lbs.

MEAL 1: Egg Scramble
4 egg whites
1 large handful spinach
½ tomato
¼ onion
1 tbsp Flax Oil
1 tbsp Smart Balance Buttery Spread with Flax Added
1 tbsp grapeseed oil

Directions:
Place pan on low-to-medium heat and grease with grapeseed oil.
Saute' chopped onion, followed by egg whites, and then spinach.
Serve topped with chopped tomato, flax oil and buttery spread.

Sides
2 slices Louis & Rich Turkey Bacon, cooked according to package directions
1 apple or pear

Drink
12oz Tropicana Orange Juice with Calcium and Vitamin D Added
1 cup Green Tea
32oz purified water

MEAL 2: Skinny Sumo Stir-fry
4oz chicken breast
2 large handfuls spinach
½ tomato
1 tbsp Flax Oil

Directions:
Sauté chicken on low-to-medium heat. In separate pan, sauté spinach until tender. Serve chicken and spinach together or separately. Top with chopped tomato and flax oil.

Sides
2 dill pickle slices
1 apple or pear

Drink
1 cup Green Tea
32oz purified water

POST WORKOUT:
30g whey protein
1 apple
½ cup dried cranberries

MEAL 4: Skinny Sumo Stir-fry

4oz chicken breast
2 large handfuls spinach
½ tomato
1 tbsp Flax Oil
1 tbsp grapeseed oil

Directions:

Sauté chicken in grapeseed oil on low-to-medium heat. In separate pan, sauté spinach until tender. Serve chicken and spinach together or separately. Top with chopped tomato and flax oil.

Sides

1 cup mixed berries
2 dill pickle slices

Drink

1 cup Green Tea
32 oz purified water

POST WORKOUT:

30g whey protein
1 cup applesauce
½ cup oatmeal

WEEK 2 • FEEDING THE FURNACE

Current weight 191.3 lbs.

6.5 lbs. down / 21.3 lbs. to go.

This week, I am slowly lowering my calories and trying to keep my food intake as low as possible, while still getting all the nutrients I need to keep me training hard. This is where the hunger bug starts talking to me.

May 17 - 23, 2007
This is the exact meal plan I followed 2 weeks before my weigh-in at 170 lbs. Any changes I have made from the previous week, I have underlined for your reference.

MEAL 1: Egg Scramble
4 egg whites
1 large handful spinach
½ tomato
¼ onion
1 tbsp Flax Oil
1 tbsp Smart Balance Buttery Spread with Flax Added
1 tbsp grapeseed oil

Directions:
Place pan on low-to-medium heat and grease with grapeseed oil. Saute' chopped onion, followed by egg whites, and then spinach. Serve topped with chopped tomato, flax oil and buttery spread.

Sides
2 slices Louis & Rich Turkey Bacon, cooked according to package directions
1 apple or pear

Drink
8oz Tropicana Orange Juice with Calcium and Vitamin D Added
1 cup Green Tea
32oz purified water

MEAL 2: Skinny Sumo Stir-fry
4oz chicken breast
2 large handfuls spinach
½ tomato
1 tbsp Flax Oil
1 tbsp grapeseed oil

Directions:
Sauté chicken in grapeseed oil on low-to-medium heat. In separate pan, sauté spinach until tender. Serve chicken and spinach together or separately. Top with chopped tomato and flax.

Sides
2 dill pickle slices
1 apple or pear

Drink
1 cup Green Tea
32oz purified water

POST WORKOUT:
20g whey protein
1 apple
½ cup dried cranberries

MEAL 4: Skinny Sumo Stir-fry
4oz chicken breast
2 large handfuls spinach
½ tomato
1 tbsp Flax Oil
1 tbsp grapeseed oil

Directions:
Sauté chicken in grapeseed oil on low-to-medium heat. In separate pan, sauté spinach until tender. Serve chicken and spinach together or separately. Top with chopped tomato and flax.

Sides
1 cup mixed berries
2 dill pickle slices

Drink
1 cup Green Tea
32oz purified water

POST WORKOUT:
20g whey protein
1 cup applesauce
½ cup oatmeal

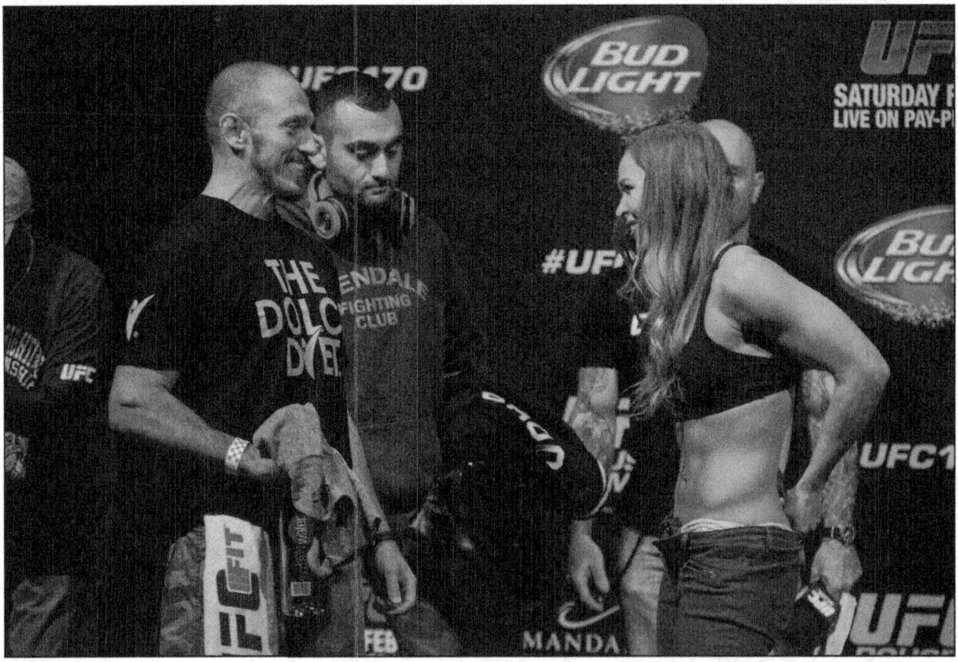

"Rowdy" Ronda Rousey gets ready to weigh in for UFC 170.

WEEK 3 • STOKING THE FLAMES

Current weight 186.2 lbs.

11.6 lbs. down / 16.2 lbs. to go

Again, I have further reduced calories and am now operating at a calorie deficit. Not the healthiest situation, but I am being monitored by my doctor and feel good. I sodium-load the first half of this week. Here, I add extra sodium to my diet, above my normal intake. This urges my body to store extra water. Don't worry, it makes sense on the next page.

Remember, any changes from the previous week are underlined.

May 24 - 27, 2007

*This is the exact meal plan I followed the first half of my weigh-in week. Any changes I have made from the previous week, I have underlined for your reference.

MEAL 1: Egg Scramble
<u>3 egg whites</u>
1 large handful spinach
<u>¼ tomato</u>
¼ onion
1 tbsp Flax Oil
1 tbsp Smart Balance Buttery Spread with Flax Added
1 tbsp grapeseed oil

Directions:
Place pan on low-to-medium heat and grease with grapeseed oil. Saute' chopped onion, followed by egg whites, and then spinach. Serve topped with chopped tomato, flax oil and buttery spread.

Sides

1 apple or pear
4 slices Louis & Rich Turkey bacon, cooked according to package directions

Drink

6oz Tropicana Orange Juice with Calcium and Vitamin D Added
1 cup Green Tea
32oz purified water

MEAL 2: Egg Scramble

3 egg whites
2 large handfuls spinach
¼ tomato
1 tbsp Flax Oil
1 tbsp Extra Virgin Olive Oil
1 tbsp grapeseed oil

Directions:

Place pan on low-to-medium heat and grease with grapeseed oil. Saute' chopped onion, followed by egg whites, and then spinach. Serve topped with chopped tomato, flax oil and buttery spread.

Sides

1 dill pickle slice
1 apple or pear

Drink

1 cup Green Tea
32oz purified water

POST WORKOUT:

15g whey protein
1 apple
½ cup dried cranberries

MEAL 4: Salmon and Veggies

4oz steamed salmon
2 large handfuls spinach
½ tomato
1 tbsp Flax Oil
1 tbsp grapeseed oil

Directions:

Sauté salmon in grapeseed oil on low-to-medium heat. In separate pan, sauté spinach until tender. Serve salmon and spinach together or separately. Top with chopped tomato and flax.

Sides

1 cup mixed berries
2 dill pickle slices

Drink

1 cup Green Tea
32oz purified water

POST WORKOUT:

15g whey protein
1 cup applesauce
0 cup oatmeal (oatmeal has been removed from tonight's menu)

FINAL 3 DAYS BEFORE WEIGH-IN

Current weight 183.4 lbs.

14.4 lbs. down / 13.4 lbs. to go

Here, I am basically running on pure motivation. The foods I am eating are keeping my blood sugar stable and getting me through training but not too much else. I have eliminated all sodium and have started drinking as much water as I can handle. I stop drinking water about 2 hours before I go to bed on the night before weigh-ins.

May 28 - 30, 2007
This is the exact meal plan I followed for this week.

MEAL 1: Egg Scramble
3 egg whites
1 large handful spinach
0 tomato (item has been removed)
0 onion (item has been removed)
1 tbsp Flax Oil
0 tbsp Smart Balance Buttery Spread with Flax Added (item has been removed)
1 tbsp grapeseed oil

Directions:
Place pan on low-to-medium heat and grease with grapeseed oil. Cook egg whites first, and then scramble with spinach. Serve topped with flax oil.

Sides
1 apple or pear
<u>0 Louis & Rich turkey bacon</u> (item has been removed)

Drink
6oz Tropicana Orange Juice with Calcium and Vitamin D Added
1 cup Green Tea
32oz purified water

MEAL 2: Egg Scramble
3 egg whites
2 large handfuls spinach
<u>0 tomato</u> (item has been removed)
1 tbsp Flax Oil
1 tbsp grapeseed oil

Directions:
Place pan on low-to-medium heat and grease with grapeseed oil. Saute' chopped onion, followed by egg whites, and then spinach. Serve topped with flax oil.

Sides
<u>0 dill pickle slice</u> (item has been removed)
1 apple or pear

Drink
1 cup Green Tea
32oz purified water

POST WORKOUT:
0g whey protein (item has been removed)
1 apple
1/2 cup dried cranberries

MEAL 4: Berry & Spinach Salad*
*(*Note: last week this was the Salmon and Veggies meal.)*
0oz steamed salmon (item has been removed)
2 large handfuls spinach
0 tomato (item has been removed)
1 cup mixed berries
1 tbsp Flax Oil
1 tbsp Extra Virgin Olive Oil

Directions:
Toss spinach with berries and top with flax and olive oil.

Sides
0 dill pickle slices (item has been removed)

Drink
1 cup Green Tea
32oz purified water

POST WORKOUT:
0g whey protein (item has been removed)
1 cup applesauce
0 cup oatmeal (item has been removed)

WEIGH-IN DAY

May 31, 2007
Wake-up weight 178.6 lbs. / 8.6 lbs. to go

Waking up today, I feel strong! Thin, but STRONG! Today, I only had 8.6 lbs. of water weight to lose. The sodium loading and depletion of this week has helped my body to naturally purge water without excessive energy expenditure.

Also, my intestinal tract is totally empty, so I do not have to cut any excess "food" weight that may be moving through my digestive system.

As is my normal weight-cut ritual, I have brewed a ¼ cup of strong coffee and grabbed a half-dollar size of dark chocolate to get my metabolism started and provide a slight boost of energy to get me through the next few hours.

I used to "hot box" much of my weight off in a sauna, but have since learned from that early mistake.

Now, I dress myself in multiple layers of sweat suits, hats and gloves and go for a brisk walk on a treadmill.

Typically, I lose an average of 1 lb. per 10 minutes, once I am warmed up and sweating.

Today, I must weigh 170 lbs., which means 90 minutes of walking.
I have learned to take my time with my weight cuts and make it as stress-free and enjoyable as possible.

With my iPod in hand and a smile on my face, I have allotted myself 180 minutes to get the weight off. The extra time will keep me calm and allow me to take a break if I need one, without feeling rushed. The worst thing that could happen is that I am done a bit early and I can shower and put on dry, clean clothes before being transported to the official venue.

There you have it - the original 3 Weeks to Shredded from 2007. So what's the difference between then and now?

A few things...

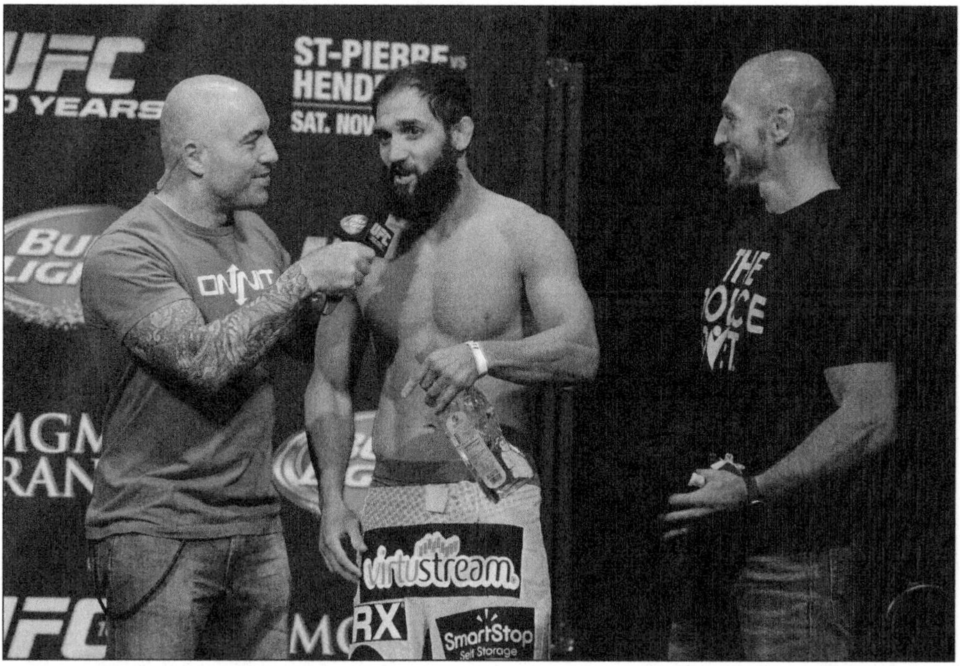

Johny Hendricks is interviewed by Joe Rogan after weighing in. Mike's athletes begin rehydrating immediately after stepping off the scale.

"Change is the law of life. And those who look only to the past or present are certain to miss the future." -John F. Kennedy

Part III

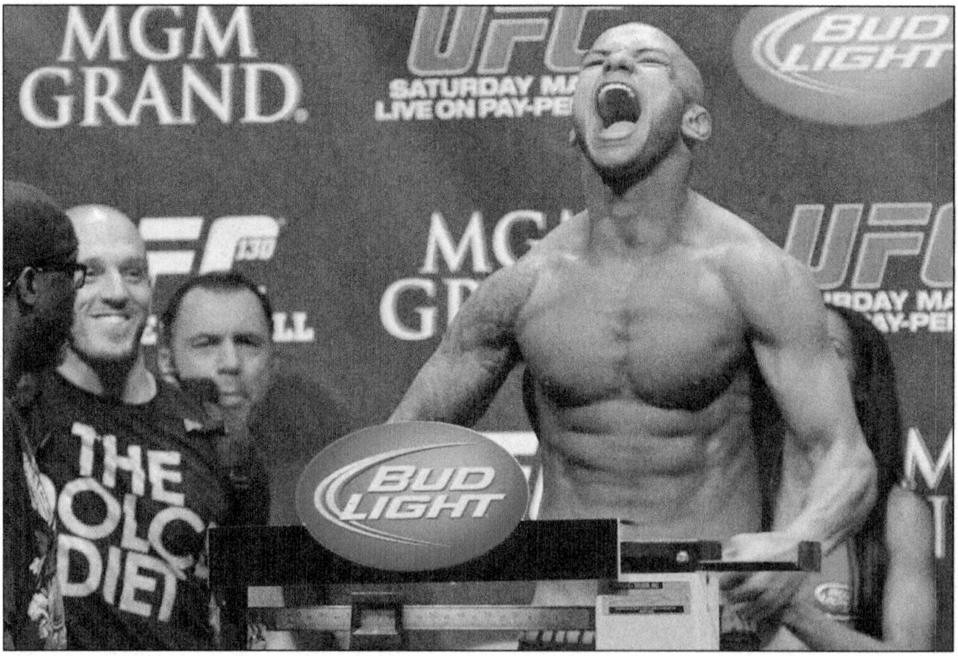

UFC welterweight Thiago "Pitbull" Alves weighs in at 170 lbs.

THE NEW 3 WEEKS TO SHREDDED

As you know, I initially wrote 3 Weeks to Shredded in 2007 based on a weight-cut technique I used at that time. Since then, I dramatically evolved the weight cut for performance.

There are many different styles and techniques that I use to temporarily shed lbs. The method is based upon the unique variables within a given situation as it pertains to an individual athlete. The following 3-Week meal plan is one of the most effective forms of weight cutting I currently use, while maintaining the healthiest possible lifestyle. As you will see, the meals I suggest are delicious; the ingredients listed are among the most nutritious on the planet.

The next chapter contains the exact program Thiago Alves followed after his 25-month layoff due to injury. On April 19, 2014, he re-emerged to win a unanimous decision victory, as well as every round on the judges' score cards. The performance also won Thiago the UFC "Fight of the Night" bonus!

HYDRATION

Each of us has our own unique hydration need. In my opinion, 1 gallon is the minimum amount of water a healthy active adult should be consuming daily. For example, I'm a 195-lb. man at 7 percent body fat. I feel and perform at my best when I drink 1.5 to 2 gallons of water per day based upon my average daily schedule. During the times I'm training harder — and specifically while cutting weight — I need more water.

The US Department of Agriculture Dietary Reference Intake Chart recommends different water intake for people based on age and sex. The USDA indicates the average adult female aged 19-to-30 years old should drink about .71 gallons of water per day, while the average 19-to-30-year-old adult male should drink .97 gallons per day. This includes water in coffee, foods, and flavored beverages, according to the USDA. In my opinion, I believe most active, healthy adults would benefit from drinking much more water, especially if they replace other processed drinks, juices and sports beverages with simple purified water.

DOLCE DIET HYDRATION PROGRAM

This is how Thiago Alves hydrated himself during fight week.

Week 1
Start at 1 gallon per day and finish the week at 1.5 gallons per day.

Week 2
Finish the week at 2 gallons per day.

Week 3
Wednesday of Week 3 we peak at 3 gallons.

On Thursday of Week 3, 1 gallon is consumed 24 hours (by 4pm Thursday in most cases) prior to weigh-ins.

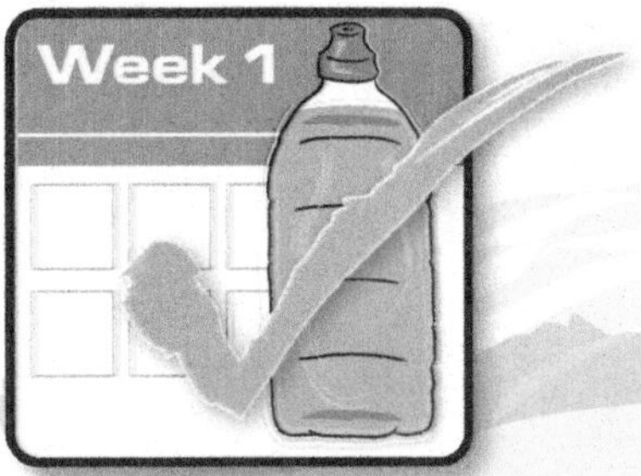

Start at 1 gallon per day and finish the week at 1.5 gallons per day.

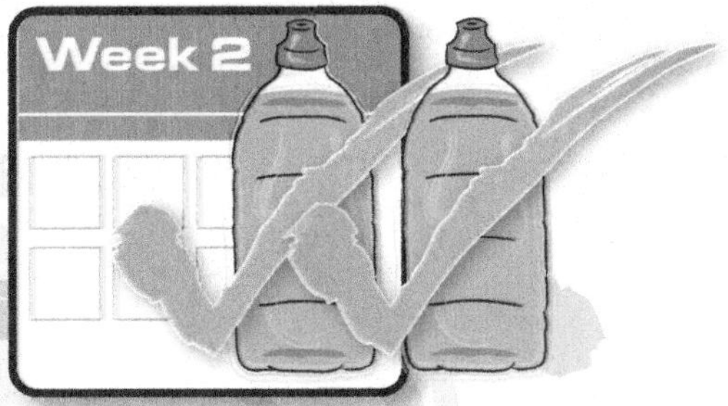

Finish the week at 2 gallons per days.

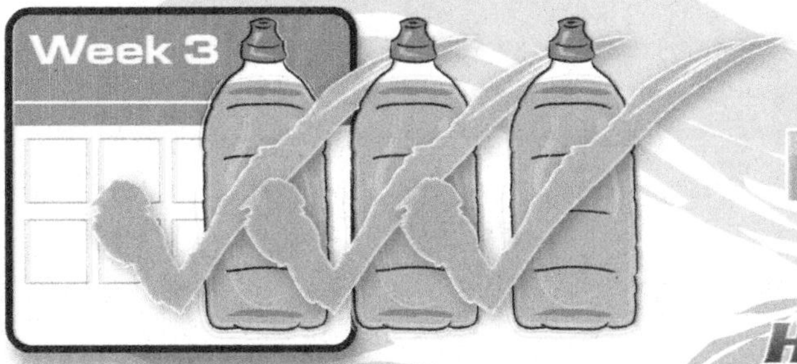

Wednesday of Week Three should peak at 3 gallons.
On Thursday of Week Three you should have one gallon consumed 24 hours prior to weigh-ins. This is 4pm Thursday in most cases.

THE DOLCE DIET Hydration

"Progress is impossible without change, and those who cannot change their minds cannot change anything." ~George Bernard Shaw

3 WEEKS TO SHREDDED: REVISED MEAL PLAN

This is the exact meal plan I used with Thiago "Pitbull" Alves' powerful, career defining comeback performance. After 2 years removed from the UFC due to injury, the Pitbull came back healthier — but thankfully not hungrier — than ever! Why? Because we fed him all the way to the scale!

All foods in this meal plan must adhere to The Dolce Diet Principles (See chapter1)

- wild caught
- organic non GMO
- fresh
- local
- minimal processing

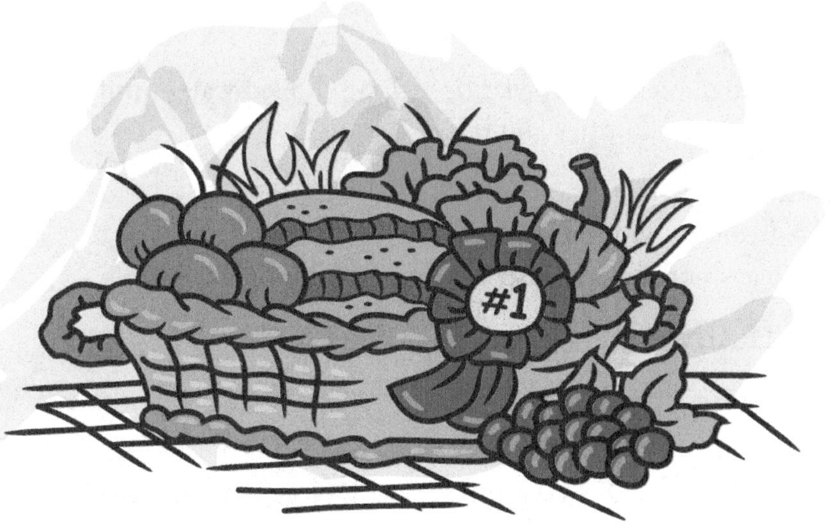

MARCH 28, 29, 30, 31
FRIDAY, SATURDAY, SUNDAY, MONDAY

STARTING WEIGHT 198 lbs.

Weigh-ins are typically on a Friday so we start the 3 Weeks to Shredded meal plan exactly 3 weeks before weigh-in day.

8:30am MEAL 1
Drink 16oz water and take 1000mg Vitamin C

Breakfast Bowl
⅓ cup oat bran
2 tbsp chia seeds
3 tbsp hemp seeds
⅓ cup raisins
1 cup mixed berries
2 tbsp almond butter
cinnamon

Directions:
Add dry ingredients to bowl. Stir in 1 cup boiled water until thickened. Top with almond butter and berries.

Drink
1 cup green tea with breakfast
1 cup black coffee with 1 tsp coconut oil after breakfast

11am TRAIN

12:30pm POST WORKOUT
30g protein*
(*Go to TheDolceDiet.com for a list of Dolce Approved protein sources.)
12oz coconut water
1 cup blueberries

1:15pm MEAL 2
16oz water with 1000mg Vitamin C

Egg Scramble
4 whole eggs
2 handfuls spinach
¼ red pepper
½ green pepper
¼ red onion
½ tomato
1 tsp avocado oil

Directions:
Grease pan with avocado oil. Scramble together above ingredients beginning with peppers and onion, then eggs. Add in spinach last. Top with chopped tomato.

Sides
3 pieces turkey bacon
1 pear

Drink
1 cup green tea
1 cup black coffee with 1 tsp coconut oil

4:30pm PRE-TRAINING SNACK
½ avocado
1 whole orange
1 cup green tea

6pm TRAIN

8pm POST WORKOUT
30g protein
12oz coconut water
1 cup blueberries

8:45pm MEAL 3
16oz water with 1000mg Vitamin C

Skinny Sumo Stir-Fry
8oz chicken
1 handful spinach
1 handful asparagus
¼ red pepper
4 cloves garlic
1 tbsp + 1 tsp avocado oil

Directions:
Cut chicken into bite-sized pieces and sauté in avocado oil.
In separate pan, sauté asparagus in 1 tsp of avocado oil. Once asparagus are tender, toss in pepper, garlic and spinach. Add vegetables and chicken together in bowl and serve.

10:30pm BEDTIME SNACK
1 apple
2 tbsp almond butter
1 square ChocoFree Metabolate

TUESDAY, APRIL 1

Note: Salad substitute for dinner

STARTING WEIGHT 194 lbs.

8:30am MEAL 1
Drink 16oz water and take 1000mg Vitamin C

Breakfast Bowl
⅓ cup oat bran
2 tbsp chia seeds
3 tbsp hemp seeds
⅓ cup raisins
1 cup mixed berries
2 tbsp almond butter
cinnamon

Directions:
Add dry ingredients to bowl. Stir in 1 cup boiled water until thickened. Top with almond butter and berries.

Drink
1 cup green tea with breakfast
1 cup black coffee with 1 tsp coconut oil after breakfast

11am TRAIN

12:30pm POST WORKOUT
30g protein
12oz coconut water
1 cup blueberries

1:15pm MEAL 2
16oz water with 1000mg Vitamin C

Egg Scramble
4 whole eggs
2 handfuls spinach
¼ red pepper
½ green pepper
¼ red onion
½ tomato
1 tsp. avocado oil

Directions:
Grease pan with avocado oil. Add in above ingredients beginning with peppers and onion, then eggs. Add in spinach last. Scramble together. Served topped with chopped tomato.

Sides
3 pieces turkey bacon
1 pear

Drinks
1 cup green tea
1 cup black coffee with 1 tsp coconut oil

4:30pm PRE-TRAINING SNACK
½ avocado
1 whole orange
1 cup green tea

6pm TRAIN

8pm POST WORKOUT
30g protein
12oz coconut water
1 cup blueberries

8:45pm MEAL 3
16oz water with 1000mg Vitamin C

The Shredded Salad
Ingredients:
1 handful spinach
1 handful kale
1 handful chopped asparagus
¼ red pepper
½ tomato
⅓ cup blue cheese crumbles
⅓ cup raisins
⅓ cup black beans
2 tbsp chia seeds
2 tbsp hemp seeds
2 tbsp extra virgin olive oil
2 tbsp balsamic vinegar to taste
⅓ cup roasted almonds drizzled in 1 tsp honey

Directions:
Toss ingredients together in large bowl and serve.

Side

⅓ cup roasted almonds drizzled with 1 tsp honey (eat on the side or add into salad)

Directions:

Sauté almonds in pan over low heat for about 2 minutes. Constantly mix them around the pan. Place almonds in small bowl and drizzle lightly with honey.

10:30pm BEDTIME SNACK

1 apple
2 tbsp almond butter
1 square ChocoFree Metabolate

WEDNESDAY, APRIL 2 (RE-FEED DAY)

STARTING WEIGHT 192 lbs.

8:30am MEAL 1

Drink 16oz water and take 1000mg Vitamin C

Breakfast Bowl

⅓ cup oat bran
2 tbsp chia seeds
3 tbsp hemp seeds
⅓ cup raisins
1 cup mixed berries
2 tbsp almond butter
cinnamon

Directions:

Add dry ingredients to bowl. Stir in 1 cup boiled water until thickened. Top with almond butter and berries.

Drink

1 cup green tea with breakfast
1 cup black coffee with 1 tsp coconut oil after breakfast

11am TRAIN

12:30pm POST WORKOUT

30g protein
12oz coconut water
1 cup blueberries

1:15pm MEAL 2
16oz water with 1000mg Vitamin C

Egg Scramble
4 whole eggs
2 handfuls spinach
¼ red pepper
½ green pepper
¼ red onion
½ tomato
1 tsp. avocado oil

Directions:
Grease pan with avocado oil and put on low-medium heat. Add in above ingredients beginning with peppers and onion, then eggs. Add in spinach last. Scramble together. Served topped with chopped tomato.

Sides
2 slices Ezekiel toast
½ avocado
3 pieces turkey bacon
1 pear

Drink
1 cup green tea
1 cup black coffee with 1 tsp coconut oil

4:30pm PRE-TRAINING SNACK
½ avocado
1 whole orange
1 cup green tea

6pm TRAIN

8pm POST WORKOUT
30g whey
12oz coconut water
1 cup blueberries

8:45pm MEAL 3
16oz water with 1000mg Vitamin C

Skinny Sumo Stir-fry
8oz chicken
1 handful spinach
1 handful asparagus
¼ red pepper
4 cloves garlic
1 tbsp + 1 tsp avocado oil

Directions:
Cut chicken into bite-sized pieces and sauté in avocado oil.
In separate pan, sauté asparagus in 1 tsp of avocado oil. Once asparagus are tender, toss in pepper, garlic and spinach. Add vegetables and chicken together in bowl and serve.

Side
⅓ cup amaranth cooked according to package directions

10:30pm BEDTIME SNACK
1 apple
2 tbsp almond butter
1 square ChocoFree Metabolate

APRIL 3, 4, 5, 6
THURSDAY, FRIDAY, SATURDAY, SUNDAY

STARTING WEIGHT 194 lbs.

8:30am MEAL 1
Drink 16oz water and take 1500mg Vitamin C

Breakfast Bowl
¼ cup oat bran
2 tbsp chia seeds
3 tbsp hemp seeds
¼ cup raisins
1 cup mixed berries
2 tbsp almond butter
cinnamon

Directions:
Add dry ingredients to bowl. Stir in 1 cup boiled water until thickened. Top with almond butter and berries.

Drink
1 cup green tea with breakfast
1 cup black coffee with 1 tsp coconut oil after breakfast

11am TRAIN

12:30pm POST WORKOUT
25g protein
12oz coconut water
1 cup blueberries

1:15pm MEAL 2
16oz water with 1500mg Vitamin C

Egg Scramble
3 whole eggs
2 handfuls spinach
¼ red pepper
½ green pepper
¼ red onion
½ tomato
1 tsp avocado oil

Directions:
Grease pan with avocado oil and put on low-medium heat. Add in above ingredients beginning with peppers and onion, then eggs. Add in spinach last. Scramble together. Served topped with chopped tomato.

Sides
2 pieces turkey bacon
1 pear

Drink
1 cup green tea
1 cup black coffee with 1 tsp coconut oil

4:30pm PRE-TRAINING SNACK
½ avocado
1 whole orange
1 cup green tea

6pm TRAIN

8pm POST WORKOUT
25g protein
12oz coconut water
1 cup blueberries

8:45pm MEAL 3
16oz water with 1500mg Vitamin C

Salmon Filet with Veggies
6oz salmon filet
1 handful spinach
1 handful asparagus
¼ red pepper
4 cloves garlic
2 tsp avocado oil

Directions:
Add 1 tsp avocado oil to pan and put on low-medium heat. Sauté asparagus until nearly tender. When asparagus is almost done add in garlic, pepper and spinach. Sauté together until tender. In separate pan, add 1 tsp avocado oil and put on low-medium heat. Cook salmon filet about 5-7 minutes until flaky. Plate and serve.

10:30pm BEDTIME SNACK
1 apple
2 tbsp almond butter
1 square ChocoFree Metabolate

MONDAY, APRIL 7

***Note:* Salad substitute for dinner**

STARTING WEIGHT 188 lbs.

8:30am MEAL 1
Drink 16oz water with 1500mg Vitamin C

Breakfast Bowl
¼ cup oat bran
2 tbsp chia seeds
3 tbsp hemp seeds
¼ cup raisins
1 cup mixed berries
2 tbsp almond butter
cinnamon

Directions:
Add dry ingredients to bowl. Stir in 1 cup boiled water until thickened. Top with almond butter and berries.

Drink
1 cup green tea with breakfast
1 cup black coffee with 1 tsp coconut oil after breakfast

11am TRAIN

12:30pm POST WORKOUT
25g protein
12oz coconut water
1 cup blueberries

1:15pm MEAL 2
16oz water with 1500mg Vitamin C

Egg Scramble
3 whole eggs
2 handfuls spinach
¼ red pepper
½ green pepper
¼ red onion
½ tomato
1 tsp avocado oil

Directions:
Grease pan with avocado oil and put on low-medium heat. Add in above ingredients beginning with peppers and onion, then eggs. Add in spinach last. Scramble together. Served topped with chopped tomato.

Sides
2 pieces turkey bacon
1 pear

Drink
1 cup green tea
1 cup black coffee with 1 tsp coconut oil

4:30pm PRE-TRAINING SNACK
½ avocado
1 whole orange
1 cup green tea

6pm TRAIN

8pm POST WORKOUT
25g protein
12oz coconut water
1 cup blueberries

8:45pm MEAL 3
16oz water with 1500mg Vitamin C

The Shredded Salad
1 handful spinach
1 handful kale
1 handful chopped asparagus
¼ red pepper
½ tomato
¼ cup blue cheese crumbles
¼ cup raisins
2 tbsp chia seeds
2 tbsp hemp seeds
2 tbsp extra virgin olive oil
2 tbsp balsamic vinegar to taste
⅓ cup roasted almonds drizzled in 1 tsp honey
*beans have been eliminated

Directions:
Toss ingredients together in large bowl and serve.

Side
⅓ cup roasted almonds drizzled with 1 tsp honey (eat on the side or add into salad)

Directions:
Sauté almonds in pan over low heat for about 2 minutes. Constantly mix them around the pan. Place almonds in small bowl and drizzle lightly with honey.

10:30pm BEDTIME SNACK
1 apple
2 tbsp almond butter
1 square ChocoFree Metabolate

TUESDAY, APRIL 8 (RE-FEED DAY)

STARTING WEIGHT 187 lbs.

8:30am MEAL 1
Drink 16oz water and take 1500mg Vitamin C

Breakfast Bowl
¼ cup oat bran
2 tbsp chia seeds
3 tbsp hemp seeds
¼ cup raisins
1 cup mixed berries
2 tbsp almond butter
cinnamon

Directions:
Add dry ingredients to bowl. Stir in 1 cup boiled water until thickened. Top with almond butter and berries.

Drink
1 cup green tea with breakfast
1 cup black coffee with 1 tsp coconut oil after breakfast

11am TRAIN

12:30pm POST WORKOUT
25g protein
12oz coconut water
1 cup blueberries

1:15pm MEAL 2
16oz water and take 1000mg Vitamin C

Egg Scramble
3 whole eggs
2 handfuls spinach
¼ red pepper
½ green pepper
¼ red onion
½ tomato
1 tsp avocado oil

Directions:
Grease pan with avocado oil and put on low-medium heat. Add in above ingredients beginning with peppers and onion, then eggs. Add in spinach last. Scramble together. Served topped with chopped tomato.

Sides
1 slice Ezekiel toast
¼ avocado
2 pieces turkey bacon
1 pear

Drink
1 cup green tea
1 cup black coffee with 1 tsp coconut oil

4:30pm PRE-TRAINING SNACK
½ avocado
1 whole orange
1 cup green tea

6pm TRAIN

8pm POST WORKOUT
25g protein
12oz coconut water
1 cup blueberries

8:45pm MEAL 3
16oz water with 1500mg Vitamin C

Salmon Filet with Veggies
6oz salmon filet
1 handful spinach
1 handful asparagus
¼ red pepper
4 cloves garlic
2 tsp avocado oil

Directions:
Add 1 tsp avocado oil to pan and put on low-medium heat. Sauté asparagus until nearly tender. When asparagus is almost done add in garlic, pepper and spinach. Sauté together until tender. In separate pan, add 1 teaspoon avocado oil and put on low-medium heat. Cook salmon filet about 5-7 minutes until flaky. Plate and serve.

Side
¼ cup amaranth cooked according to package directions

10:30pm BEDTIME SNACK
1 apple
2 tbsp almond butter
1 square ChocoFree Metabolate

APRIL 9, 10, 11
WEDNESDAY, THURSDAY, FRIDAY

STARTING WEIGHT 187 lbs.

8:30am MEAL 1
Drink 16oz water and take 2000mg Vitamin C

Breakfast Bowl
¼ cup oat bran
2 tbsp chia seeds
3 tbsp hemp seeds
¼ cup raisins
1 cup mixed berries
2 tbsp almond butter
dash of cinnamon
¼ tsp Pink Himalayan sea salt

Directions:
Add dry ingredients to bowl. Stir in 1 cup boiled water until thickened. Top with almond butter and berries.

Drink
1 cup green tea with breakfast
1 cup black coffee with 1 tsp coconut oil after breakfast

11am TRAIN

12:30pm POST WORKOUT
20g protein
4oz applesauce

1:15pm MEAL 2
16oz water with 2000mg Vitamin C

Egg Scramble
2 whole eggs
2 handfuls spinach
¼ red pepper
½ green pepper
¼ red onion
¼ tomato
1 tbsp. avocado oil
¼ tsp Pink Himalayan sea salt

Directions:
Add 1 teaspoon avocado oil to pan and put on low-medium heat. Add in above ingredients beginning with peppers and onion, then eggs. Add in spinach last. Scramble together. Served topped with chopped tomato.

Sides
3 pieces turkey bacon
1 apple

Drink
1 cup green tea
1 cup black coffee with 1 tsp coconut oil

4:30pm PRE-TRAINING SNACK
¼ avocado
½ an orange
1 cup green tea

6pm TRAIN

8pm POST WORKOUT
20g protein
4oz applesauce

8:45pm MEAL 3
16oz water with 2000mg Vitamin C

Salmon Filet with Veggies
4oz salmon filet
1 handful spinach
1 handful asparagus
¼ red pepper
4 cloves garlic
2 tsp. avocado oil
¼ tsp Pink Himalayan sea salt

Directions:
Add 1 teaspoon avocado oil to pan and put on low-medium heat. Sauté asparagus until nearly tender. When asparagus is almost done add in garlic, pepper and spinach. Sauté together until tender. In separate pan, add 1 teaspoon avocado oil and put on low-medium heat. Cook salmon filet about 5-7 minutes until flaky. Plate and serve.

10:30pm BEDTIME SNACK
1 apple
2 tbsp almond butter
1 square ChocoFree Metabolate

SATURDAY, APRIL 12 *PROTEIN PARTY

STARTING WEIGHT 188 lbs.

8:30am MEAL 1
Drink 16oz water and take 2000mg Vitamin C

Breakfast Bowl
¼ cup oat bran
2 tbsp chia seeds
3 tbsp hemp seeds
¼ cup raisins
1 cup mixed berries
2 tbsp almond butter
cinnamon
¼ tsp Pink Himalayan sea salt

Directions:
Add dry ingredients to bowl. Stir in 1 cup boiled water until thickened. Top with almond butter and berries.

Drink
1 cup green tea with breakfast
1 cup black coffee with 1 tsp coconut oil after breakfast

11am TRAIN

12:30pm POST WORKOUT
20g protein
4oz applesauce

1:15pm MEAL 2
16oz water with 2000mg Vitamin C

Egg Scramble
2 whole eggs
2 handfuls spinach
¼ red pepper
½ green pepper
¼ red onion
¼ tomato
1 tsp avocado oil
¼ tsp Pink Himalayan sea salt

Directions:
Grease pan with avocado oil and put on low-medium heat. Add in ingredients beginning with peppers and onion, then eggs. Add in spinach last. Scramble together. Serve topped with chopped tomato.

Sides
3 pieces turkey bacon
1 apple

Drink
1 cup green tea
1 cup black coffee with 1 tsp coconut oil

4:30pm PRE-TRAINING SNACK
¼ avocado
½ an orange
1 cup green tea

6pm TRAIN

8pm POST WORKOUT
20g protein
4oz applesauce

8:45pm MEAL 3
16oz water with 2000mg Vitamin C

***Steak with Veggies**
12oz grass-fed steak
1 handful spinach
1 handful asparagus
¼ red pepper
4 cloves garlic
2 tsp. avocado oil
¼ tsp Pink Himalayan sea salt

Directions:
Preheat oven to 400 F. Add 1 teaspoon avocado oil to pan and put on low-medium heat. Sauté asparagus until nearly tender. When asparagus is almost done add in garlic, pepper and spinach. Sauté together until tender. In separate pan, add 1 teaspoon avocado oil and put on medium heat. Sear steak about 1 minute on each side. Place in glass baking dish and put in oven for 10-15 minutes depending on thickness. Once cooked to your taste, remove steak from oven and serve with vegetables.

10:30pm BEDTIME SNACK
1 apple
2 tbsp almond butter
1 square ChocoFree Metabolate

SUNDAY, APRIL 13

STARTING WEIGHT 188 lbs.

10am WAKE

MODIFIED FAST

Drink 32oz water within the first 30 minutes of waking up.
Take 3000mg Vitamin C / 1500mg Dandelion Root / 1500mg Uva Ursi
Follow with green tea mixed with 1 tbsp honey and 1 cup black coffee mixed with 1 tsp coconut oil

1:15pm MEAL 1

16oz water with 3000mg Vitamin C / 1500mg Dandelion Root / 1500mg Uva Ursi

Egg Scramble

2 whole eggs
1 handful spinach
¼ red pepper
¼ red onion
¼ tomato
1 tsp avocado oil

Directions:

Grease pan with avocado oil and put on low-medium heat. Add in above ingredients beginning with peppers and onion, then eggs. Add in spinach last. Scramble together. Served topped with chopped tomato.

Side

1 apple

Drink
1 cup green tea with breakfast
1 cup black coffee with 1 tsp coconut oil after breakfast

4:30pm SNACK

¼ avocado
½ an orange
1 cup green tea

7:30pm MEAL 2

16oz water with 3000mg Vitamin C / 1500mg Dandelion Root / 1500mg Uva Ursi

Skinny Sumo Stir-fry
4 oz chicken
1 handful asparagus
¼ red pepper
4 cloves garlic
1 tbsp + 1 tsp avocado oil

Directions:
Cut chicken into bite-sized pieces and sauté in avocado oil. In separate pan, sauté asparagus in 1 tsp of avocado oil. Once asparagus are tender, toss in pepper, garlic and spinach. Add vegetables and chicken together in bowl and serve.

10:30pm BEDTIME SNACK

1 apple
2 tbsp raw, unsalted almond butter
1 square ChocoFree Metabolate

MONDAY, APRIL 14

STARTING WEIGHT 185 lbs.

8:30am BREAKFAST
16oz water with 3000mg Vitamin C / 1500mg Dandelion Root / 1500mg Uva Ursi

Breakfast Bowl
¼ cup oat bran
2 tbsp chia seeds
2 tbsp hemp seeds
¼ cup raisins
½ cup mixed berries
1 tbsp unsalted almond butter
cinnamon

Directions:
Add dry ingredients to bowl. Stir in 1 cup boiled water until thickened. Top with almond butter and berries.

Drink
1 cup green tea with breakfast
1 cup black coffee with 1 tsp coconut oil after breakfast

10:30am-11:30am TRAIN: Treadmill
15 minute walk at 3.5mph
30 minute jog at 5.5mph
15 minute walk at 3.5mph

12:30pm LUNCH
16oz water with 3000mg Vitamin C / 1500mg Dandelion Root / 1500mg Uva Ursi

Egg Scramble
2 whole eggs
1 handful spinach
¼ red pepper
¼ red onion
¼ tomato
1 tsp avocado oil

Directions:
Grease pan with avocado oil and put on low-medium heat. Add in above ingredients beginning with peppers and onion, then eggs. Add in spinach last. Scramble together. Served topped with chopped tomato.

Side
1 apple

Drink
1 cup green tea
1 cup black coffee with 1 tsp coconut oil

4:30pm SNACK
16oz water with 3000mg Vitamin C / 1500mg Dandelion Root / 1500mg Uva Ursi
¼ avocado
½ an orange
1 cup green tea

6:30pm-7:30pm PERFORM DOLCE STEP METHOD / HOT TUB

8pm DINNER
16oz water with 3000mg Vitamin C / 1500mg Dandelion Root / 1500mg Uva Ursi

Egg Scramble (Or Cold Salad*)
2 whole eggs
1 handful spinach
½ handful kale
½ tomato
¼ red pepper
¼ red onion
2 tbsp chia seeds
2 tbsp hemp seeds
1 tsp. avocado oil

Directions:
Add 1 teaspoon avocado oil to pan and put on low-medium heat. Add in ingredients beginning with red pepper and onion, then eggs. Add in spinach and kale. Mix in chia and hemp seeds. Scramble together. Serve topped with chopped tomato.

*To make the cold salad: Add all ingredients except eggs to a large bowl. Scramble eggs and place atop salad.

Side
⅓ cup roasted almonds drizzled with 1 tsp honey (can add to salad)

Directions:
Sauté almonds in pan over low heat for about 2 minutes.

Constantly mix them around the pan. Place almonds in small bowl and drizzle lightly with honey.

10:30pm BEDTIME SNACK

1 apple
1 tbsp unsalted almond butter
1 square ChocoFree Metabolate

TUESDAY, APRIL 15

STARTING WEIGHT 183 lbs.

8:30am BREAKFAST
16oz water with 3000mg Vitamin C / 1500mg Dandelion Root / 1500mg Uva Ursi

Breakfast Bowl
¼ cup oat bran
2 tbsp chia seeds
2 tbsp hemp seeds
¼ cup raisins
½ cup mixed berries
1 tbsp unsalted almond butter
cinnamon

Directions:
Add dry ingredients to bowl. Stir in 1 cup boiled water until thickened. Top with almond butter and berries.

Drink
1 cup green tea with breakfast
1 cup black coffee with 1 tsp coconut oil after breakfast

10:30am-11:30am TRAIN: Treadmill
15 minute walk at 3.5mph
30 minute jog at 5.5mph
15 minute walk at 3.5mph

12:30pm LUNCH
16oz water with 3000mg Vitamin C / 1500mg Dandelion Root / 1500mg Uva Ursi

Egg Scramble
2 whole eggs
1 handful spinach
¼ red pepper
¼ red onion
¼ tomato
1 tsp avocado oil

Directions:
Add 1 teaspoon avocado oil to pan and put on low-medium heat. Add in ingredients beginning with red pepper and onion, then eggs. Add in spinach last. Scramble together. Serve topped with chopped tomato.

Side
1 apple

Drink
1 cup green tea
1 cup black coffee with 1 tsp coconut oil

4:30pm SNACK
16oz water with 3000mg Vitamin C / 1500mg Dandelion Root / 1500mg Uva Ursi
¼ avocado
½ an orange
1 cup green tea

6:30pm-7:30pm PERFORM DOLCE STEP METHOD / HOT TUB

8pm DINNER
16oz water with 3000mg Vitamin C / 1500mg Dandelion Root / 1500mg Uva Ursi

Egg Scramble (or Cold Salad*)
2 whole eggs
1 handful spinach
½ handful kale
½ tomato
¼ red pepper
¼ red onion
2 tbsp chia seeds
2 tbsp hemp seeds
1 tsp avocado oil

Directions:
Add 1 teaspoon avocado oil to pan and put on low-medium heat. Add in ingredients beginning with red pepper and onion, then eggs. Add in spinach and kale. Mix in chia and hemp seeds. Scramble together. Serve topped with chopped tomato.

*To make the cold salad: Add all ingredients except eggs to a large bowl. Scramble eggs and place atop salad.

10:30pm BEDTIME SNACK
1 apple
1 tbsp unsalted almond butter
1 square ChocoFree Metabolate

WEDNESDAY, APRIL 16

STARTING WEIGHT 181 lbs.

8:30am BREAKFAST
16oz water with 3000mg Vitamin C / 1500mg Dandelion Root / 1500mg Uva Ursi

Breakfast Bowl
¼ cup oat bran
2 tbsp chia seeds
2 tbsp hemp seeds
¼ cup raisins
½ cup mixed berries
1 tbsp unsalted almond butter
cinnamon

Directions:
Add dry ingredients to bowl. Stir in 1 cup boiled water until thickened. Top with almond butter and berries.

Drink
1 cup green tea with breakfast
1 cup black coffee with 1 tsp coconut oil after breakfast

10:30am-11:30am TRAIN: Treadmill
15 minute walk at 3.5mph
30 minute jog at 5.5mph
15 minute walk at 3.5mph

12:30pm LUNCH
16oz water with 3000mg Vitamin C / 1500mg Dandelion Root / 1500mg Uva Ursi

Egg Scramble
2 whole eggs
1 handful spinach
¼ red pepper
¼ red onion
¼ tomato
1 tsp avocado oil

Directions:
Add 1 teaspoon avocado oil to pan and put on low-medium heat. Add in ingredients beginning with red pepper and onion, then eggs. Add in spinach last. Scramble together. Serve topped with chopped tomato.

Side
1 apple

Drink
1 cup green tea
1 cup black coffee with 1 tsp coconut oil

4:30pm SNACK
16oz water with 3000mg Vitamin C / 1500mg Dandelion Root / 1500mg Uva Ursi
¼ avocado
½ orange
1 cup green tea

6:30pm-7:30pm PERFORM DOLCE STEP METHOD / HOT TUB

8pm DINNER
16oz water with 3000mg Vitamin C / 1500mg Dandelion Root / 1500mg Uva Ursi

Egg Scramble (or Cold Salad*)
2 whole eggs
1 handful spinach
½ handful kale
½ tomato
¼ red pepper
¼ red onion
2 tbsp chia seeds
2 tbsp hemp seeds
1 tsp avocado oil

Directions:
Add 1 teaspoon avocado oil to pan and put on low-medium heat. Add in ingredients beginning with red pepper and onion, then eggs. Add in spinach and kale. Mix in chia and hemp seeds. Scramble together. Serve topped with chopped tomato.

*To make the cold salad: Add all ingredients except eggs to a large bowl. Scramble eggs in avocado oil and place atop salad.

10:30pm BEDTIME SNACK
1 apple
1 tbsp unsalted almond butter
1 square ChocoFree Metabolate

THURSDAY, APRIL 17

STARTING WEIGHT 179 lbs.

8:30am BREAKFAST
16oz water with 3000mg Vitamin C / 1500mg Dandelion Root / 1500mg Uva Ursi

Breakfast Bowl
¼ cup oat bran
2 tbsp chia seeds
2 tbsp hemp seeds
¼ cup raisins
½ cup mixed berries
1 tbsp unsalted almond butter
cinnamon

Directions:
Add dry ingredients to bowl. Stir in 1 cup boiled water until thickened. Top with almond butter and berries.

Drink
1 cup green tea with breakfast
1 cup black coffee with 1 tsp coconut oil after breakfast

10:30am-11:30am TRAIN: Treadmill
15 minute walk at 3.5mph
30 minute jog at 5.5mph
15 minute walk at 3.5mph

12:30pm LUNCH
16oz water with 3000mg Vitamin C / 1500mg Dandelion Root / 1500mg Uva Ursi

Egg Scramble
2 whole eggs
1 handful spinach
¼ red pepper
¼ red onion
¼ tomato
1 tsp avocado oil

Directions:
Add 1 teaspoon avocado oil to pan and put on low-medium heat. Add in ingredients beginning with red pepper and onion, then eggs. Add in spinach last. Scramble together. Serve topped with chopped tomato.

Side
1 apple

Drink
1 cup green tea
1 cup black coffee with 1 tsp coconut oil

4:30pm SNACK
16oz water with 3000mg Vitamin C / 1500mg Dandelion Root / 1500mg Uva Ursi
¼ avocado
½ an orange
1 cup green tea

8pm DINNER
16oz water with 3000mg Vitamin C / 1500mg Dandelion Root / 1500mg Uva Ursi

Cold Salad
2 whole eggs
1 handful spinach
½ handful kale
½ tomato
¼ red pepper
¼ red onion
2 tbsp chia seeds
2 tbsp hemp seeds
¼ cup raisins
1 tsp avocado oil

Directions:
Add all ingredients except eggs to a large bowl. Scramble eggs in avocado oil and place atop salad.

9pm-10pm PERFORM DOLCE STEP METHOD / HOT TUB

10:30pm BEDTIME SNACK
1 apple
1 tbsp unsalted almond butter
1 square ChocoFree Metabolate

Each day of fight week, Thiago lost 2 lbs.

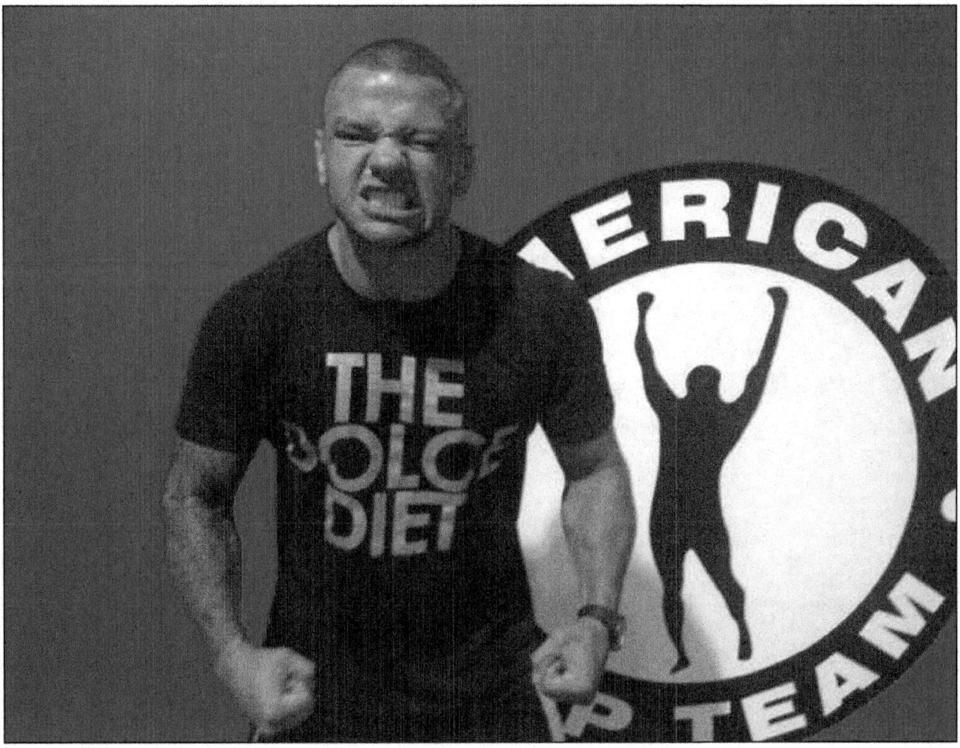

"You mess with my meals, you mess with my emotions!" Thiago Alves gets his game face on.

"The fight is won or lost far away from witnesses - behind the lines, in the gym, and out there on the road, long before I dance under those lights." *~Muhammad Ali*

WATER INTAKE DURING FIGHT WEEK

Monday 185 lbs.
- 2 gallons

Tuesday 183 lbs.
- 2.5 gallons

Wednesday 181 lbs.
- 3 gallons

Thursday 179 lbs.
- 1 gallon before noon

THURSDAY, APRIL 17 (THE DAY BEFORE WEIGH-INS)

Thiago weighed 171 lbs. when he stepped out of the hot tub at 10pm. Expecting this, I made him an 8 oz. grass-fed steak, 4 oz. sautéed spinach, and he drank 16 oz. water.

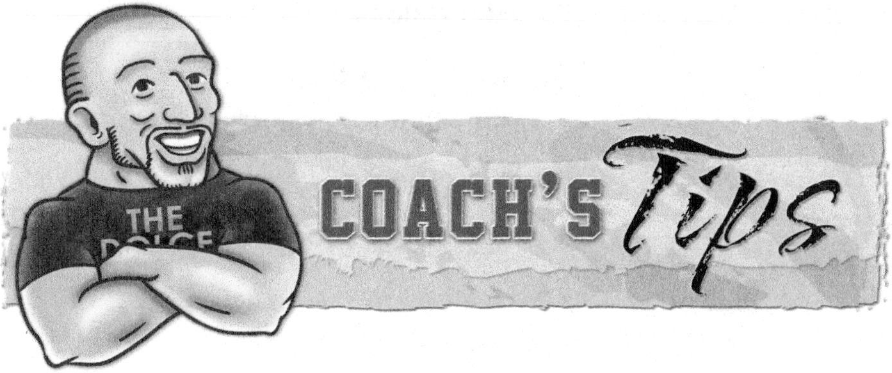

The day before weigh-ins: From this point, we eat sensibly. We don't starve ourselves, nor are we afraid to cleanse our systems and purify our bodies. We've been eating perfectly for weeks now, specifically the last 3 weeks. Our meals have become much more efficient, much cleaner. Over the next 24 hours, each ounce that we consume must be lost, so we must choose wisely. Personally, I enjoy grazing. I have no problem grabbing a few leaves of spinach and a handful of blueberries as casually as most would grab for a handful of popcorn. Today should be about relaxation, breaking small sweats without working to do so. Laying in a warm room, watching a favorite movie with their significant other happens much more often with my athletes than any of you would ever believe.

FRIDAY, APRIL 18 (WEIGH-IN DAY)

Thiago went to bed on Thursday weighing 173 lbs. and woke up Friday morning (weigh-in day) at 171.8 lbs. I gave him a 4 oz. cup of black coffee mixed with 1 teaspoon of coconut oil. We made a modified breakfast bowl: 2 tablespoons oat bran, 2 tablespoons chia seeds, 2 tablespoons hemp seeds, 2 tablespoons raisins, 1 tablespoon honey, mixed with 4 oz. boiled water. This weighed a total of 8 oz.

We had 6 hours until weigh-ins. Knowing how Thiago's body normally "floats" or loses weight during the day, we felt no need to prepare a "weight-cutting session." Within 2 trips to the restroom over the next two hours Thiago was back to 171 lbs. with hours to spare. He would sip on black coffee with coconut oil and purified water throughout the day, keeping his weight below 171.5 lbs. After one more trip to the restroom, by the time he stepped on the scale for the official UFC weigh-ins, he weighed the championship weight of 170 lbs. looking fresh and healthy!

WEIGH-IN DAY

We need our strength to endure the challenges before us, and there is no better way to start than with the breakfast bowl. It may be a little smaller than usual, maybe even just a few spoonfuls, but it's there, it's ready and it's up to the athlete how much they need to feel good.

I also make sure there's fruit readily available that the athlete can feel free to graze on at any time. So even while cutting weight, my athletes continue to consume, which helps them to maintain a vibrant level of health and strength. Because we've prepared properly, my athletes usually weigh no more than 5 lbs. above their weight class on the morning of weigh-ins. At the elite level, even on weigh-in day, the athlete has media obligations and responsibilities related to the event. Typically, my athlete wakes up at 9am. We calibrate his or her weight with the official scale as well as our personal scale to leave zero room for error.

It's important to bring your own scale with you.
Don't be afraid to spend $100 or more on your own scale. Missing weight as a professional can cause a 20 percent penalty against your purse. For that amount of money, you could've bought many scales and maintained your reputation.

Remember, my athletes are no more than 5 lbs. over on the morning of weigh-ins. Therefore, following my **Step Method** previously outlined, we can make weight within an hour's time and begin the process rehydrating often before the athlete even steps on the scale.

How do we do this? Usually, we have to meet the event coordinator at 2pm to be transported to the weigh-in venue. This means we have to be done cutting weight at 1:30pm at the latest so the athlete can shower, change, tend to any last minute needs and be the professional athlete he is by being on time. This means the athlete spends a minimum of 2 hours being "on weight." That is simply 2 hours too long. To adjust for this, I bring my scale with me and weigh my athlete every 15-30 minutes throughout the day to make sure they don't continue losing weight. If so, we immediately rehydrate or eat to maintain the weight class limit - no higher and no lower. One tool I use to keep them hydrated throughout the process is my Natural Electrolyte Drink.

At the athlete's discretion, they can also chew on our pre-planned assortment of fresh fruit including watermelon, cantaloupe, kiwi, grapes, strawberries, blueberries, raspberries, etc. To ensure we aren't overfeeding or over-drinking, I have the athlete stand on the scale and hold in his hands the amount of food and/or drink he is about to consume.

MIKE DOLCE'S NATURAL ELECTROLYTE DRINK

This drink allows you to avoid all the unnecessary sugars that famous, namebrand sports drinks contain while consuming much more electrolytes.

Ingredients
24oz room temperature water
Half a fresh-squeezed lemon
1 tbsp chia seeds
1 tbsp honey
Dash of sea salt

Directions
Mix together & drink fresh.

Nutrition Facts:
1/2 juice of lemon: 8 calories, 0 g protein, 3 g CHO, 0.1 g fat, 1 g fiber, 1 mg sodium, 40 mg potassium, 8 mg calcium, 2 mg magnesium
1 tbsp Chia Seeds: 69 calories, 2 g protein, 6 g CHO, 4.5 g fat, 1 g sat. fat, 5 g fiber, 2 mg sodium, 58 mg potassium, 89 mg calcium, 47 mg magnesium
1 tbsp honey: 64 calories, 0 g protein, 17 g CHO, 0 g fat, 0 g fiber, 1 mg sodium, 11 mg potassium, 1 mg calcium, 0 mg magnesium

Benefits:
Lemon: Packed with vitamin C to benefit skin (synthesizes production of collagen fibers to repair damaged tissue) and immune health

Chia Seeds*: Member of the mint family, excellent source of Omega-3s, fiber, protein and minerals. May help improve cardiovascular risk factors, such as, lowering cholesterol, triglycerides and blood pressure.

Honey:
Boosts immune system due to high vitamin/mineral content, naturally sweet. Aids in indigestion due to the antiseptic properties of honey and relieves acidity in the stomach.

****Academy of Nutrition and Dietetics***

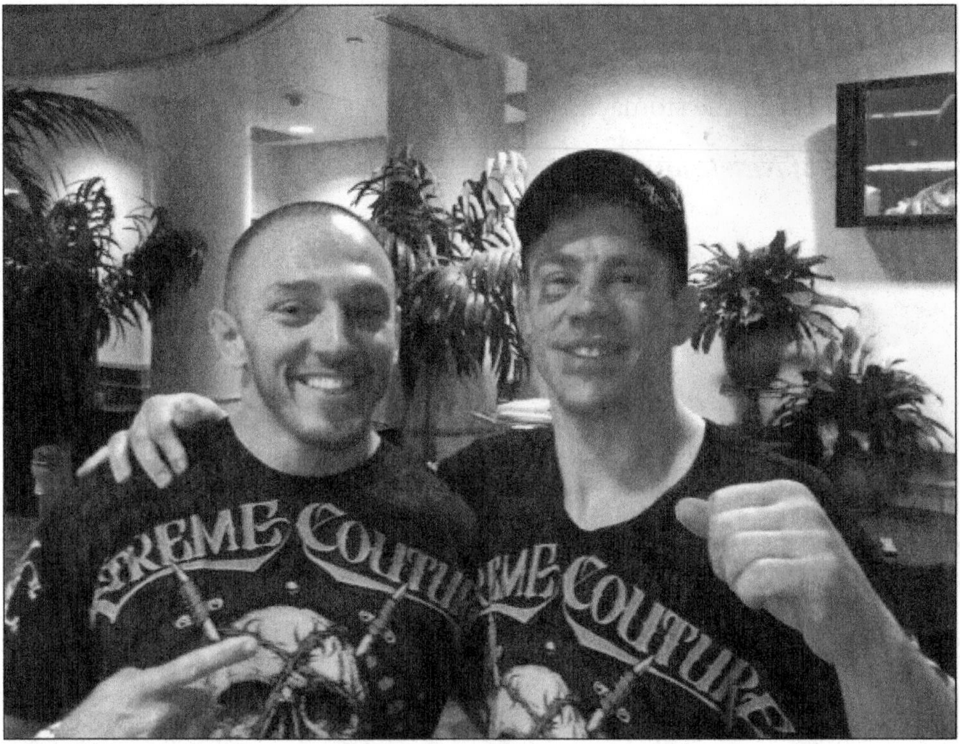

Mike Dolce and Duane "Bang" Ludwig after Ludwig defeated Amir Sadollah by unanimous decision at UFC Live 5 on Aug. 14, 2011.

Part IV

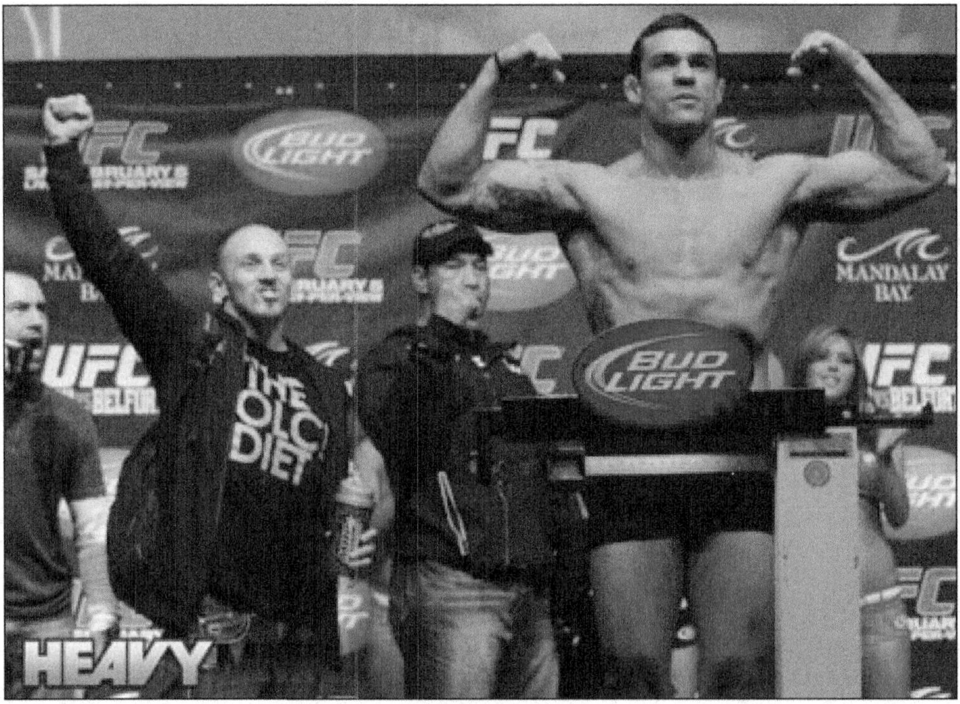

Vitor Belfort weighs in for UFC 126 via The Dolce Diet.

SAME DAY WEIGH-INS

There's been ample controversy regarding weight cuts, whether the process is healthy. The fact is that losing a great amount of weight in a short period of time is not healthy. I've always maintained this.

For the last 25 years - yes, I'm getting old - I have been cutting weight as an amateur wrestler, nationally ranked powerlifter, amateur boxer and professional mixed martial artist. I've also participated in the weight cut process thousands of times with my teammates, students and athletes. My opinion is based on personal experience tempered with all known scientific research.

My methods are here to make this process as healthy as humanly possible.

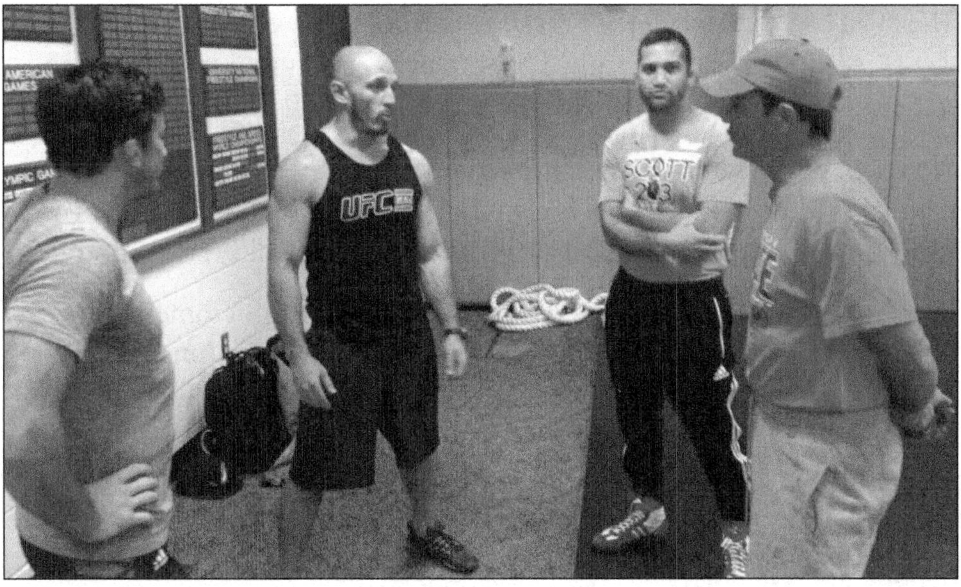

Mike Dolce speaks with (from left) 2012 Olympic Freestyle Wrestling Bronze Medalist, and 3 Weeks to Shredded user, Coleman Scott; two-time Olympic Freestyle Wrestling Gold Medalist and Oklahoma State head coach John Smith; and NCAA Division I National Champion and Oklahoma State assistant wrestling coach Zack Esposito.

Some suggest that same-day weigh-ins would be a healthier approach to two opponents being evenly matched. The fact remains, that any way you look at this situation athletes are still cutting weight. With same-day weigh-ins, the athlete will likely cut the same amount of weight and go to drastic measures to rehydrate in time for competition.

Cutting weight is not suggested for same-day competition. Think about what is healthier: 24 hours to rehydrate, or 4 hours at most? Aside from the very important aspect of maintaining health, we want to ensure optimal performance. Therefore, whether one is doing same-day weigh-ins or day-of, the approach is the same.

The most healthful way to approach both same-day weigh-ins and day-before weigh-ins is to reduce your bodyweight during training camp to be closer to your competitive weight.

However, with a same-day weigh-in competition, the fighter should be fighting as close to his natural body weight as possible. Without the overnight time to replenish the body, your performance could very well suffer.

You should be at your competitive weight comfortably for same-day weigh-ins. This way, you will ensure ample strength, energy and the ability to execute your technique.

Should you attempt to cut a similar amount of weight for a same-day weigh-in as you would a day-prior weigh-in, you will not compete up to your potential and can only hope for victory if your evenly matched opponent did it worse.

For the best chance of performing up to your greatest potential, begin the weight-loss process as soon as the competition is scheduled. Reduce body fat to the necessary point that you are simply within a bowel movement

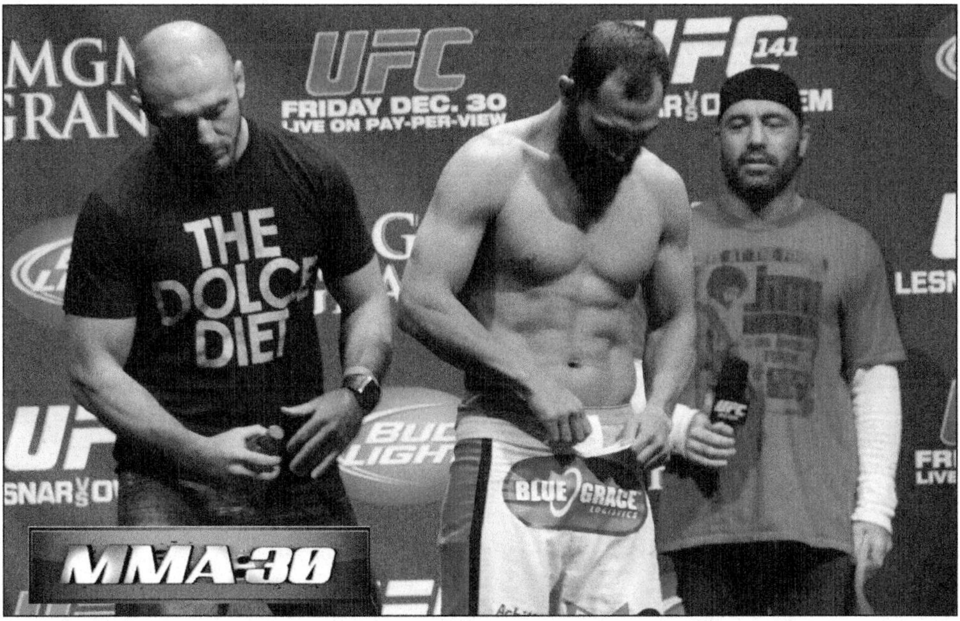

Johny "Bigg Rigg" Hendricks gets ready to weigh in for UFC 141.

of your weight-class on competition day. The preferred general body fat ratio for combat is 7-10 percent for healthy adult males (16-20 percent for healthy adult females).

Avoid foods high in sodium as they could make you hold water. Beyond that, we need to only consume foods of maximum absorption and avoid any foods that do not offer complete nourishment and aid in efficient digestion. Think lean and green! Stay away from foods that are fried, heavy in dairy, and most preserved products. In general, water is most important, as well as electrolytes.

Ultimately, it is best to not cut weight at all. You cannot retain much useable energy or any size advantage in such a short window of time. It's best to be full of 'piss and vinegar' when you step on the battlefield.

CHASE GENTLE

Starting weight: 201 lbs. • Ending weight: 190 lbs.

I kickstarted my new lifestyle with 3 Weeks to Shredded and then after 3 1/2 weeks, I switched over to Living Lean and Living Lean Cookbook. I have been weightlifting for several years now and within those years I have experimented with many different diets and workout programs. I had a buddy who told me about this diet program called, "3 Weeks to Shredded." For some reason I was mostly intrigued by the fact that you could not purchase this book anywhere but from Mike Dolce's website. I thought to myself, "Who does that these days with Amazon around?" But nonetheless I respected it greatly, because I knew whoever Mike Dolce was; he was out to help people and not to collect money.

I started the program fluctuating between 199-201 lbs. and coming off a bad diet of Monster Energy drinks and processed foods that has a longer shelf life than the plastic it was contained in. I read through the book, went shopping, and began my new lifestyle.

My goal and biggest motivation was to be lean and as ripped as possible by summer and then continue to live lean everyday. The results I saw in the mirror and the way I functioned at work (corporate America sales) were what kept me motivated through the lifestyle change.

The hardest parts were going through the headaches, sugar cravings, and withdrawals from all the crap food I lived off of previously. After about a week of my body taking in only organic Earth-grown nutrients; I started to feel better, think more clearly, have more energy and sleep better. I even monitored my sleep with a new band I wear that tracks the quality of my sleep. And I can tell you my sleep was deeper and more refreshing.

I would compare it to putting low grade fuel in a Ferrari and running it for several years and then replacing it with pure high-octane fuel and feeling the power it was originally meant to have.

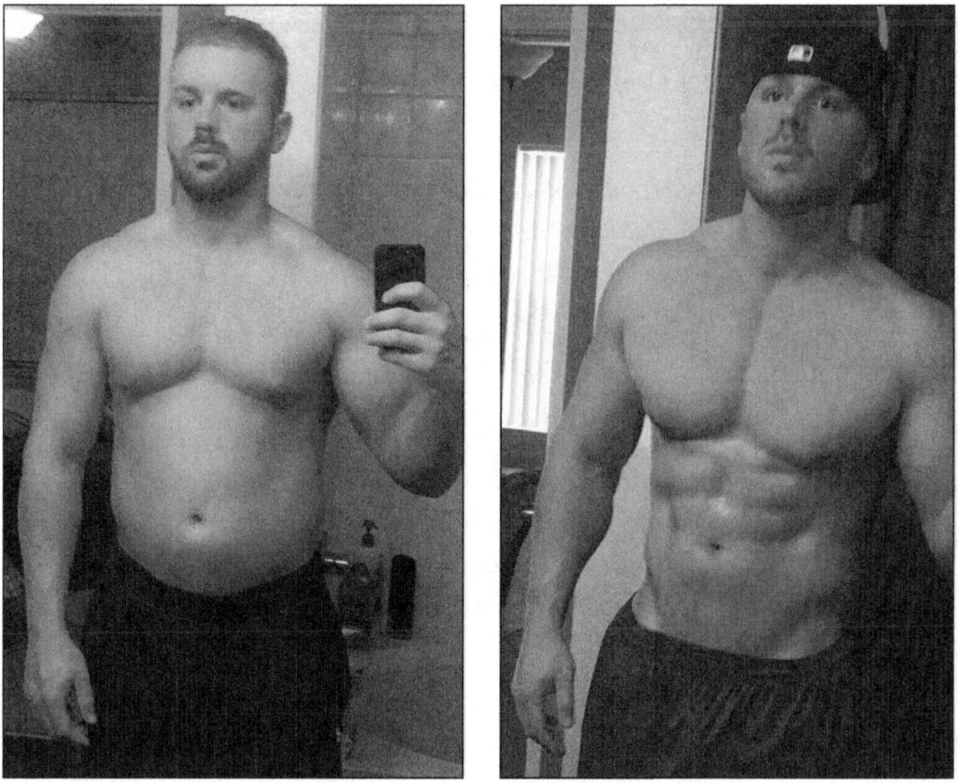

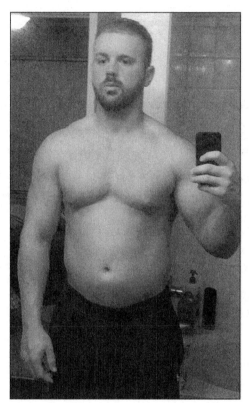

Chase Gentle before The Dolce Diet at 201 lbs. and after at 190 lbs.

I followed the diet precisely only substituting the whey protein for (a vegan-based plant protein supplement), which was only due to me having access to Mike's podcast.

My workout regiment was more of a 3-week cycle between High Intensity Interval Training, slow isolation, and bodyweight lifts; and I have continued that today as it has produced great results.

The advice I would give to someone starting this would be stick to your guns and you will have results...end of story. (Oh, and also find Mike's recipe for the Breakfast Bowl because that is a life saver!)

Thanks Mike and Brandy for all you do with Living Lean and your podcast. I am a husband and proud father of a 9-month-old who will now grow up with Earth-grown nutrients and thinking that Mike Dolce is a distant uncle who gives dad good advice! EXCUSES OR RESULTS....NOT BOTH! #BOOM

"Courage - you develop courage by doing small things like just as if you wouldn't want to pick up a 100-pound weight without preparing yourself." ~*Maya Angelou*

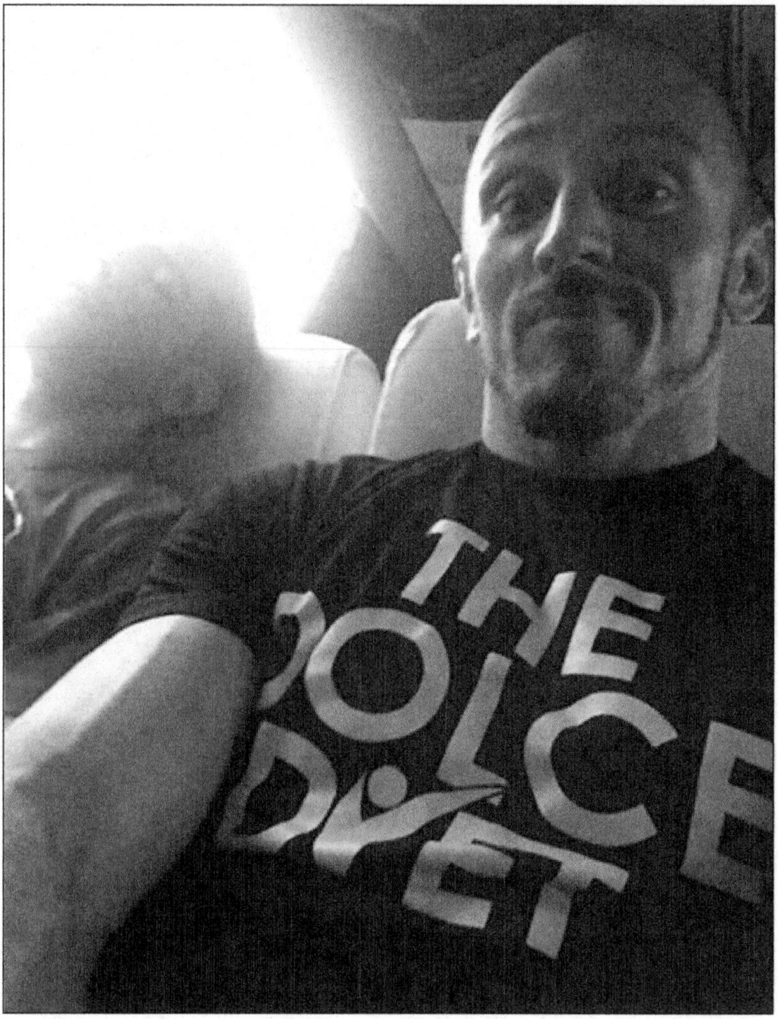

Jaragua do Sul, Santa Catarina, Brazil: Mike Dolce and a relaxing Nik Lentz make the long bus trip from the fighter hotel to weigh-ins. Often, weight cuts must be made in countries where certain "fight week" foods are unavailable. Mike always is prepared and brings essential ingredients with him.

WEIGHT-CUT DANGERS: SAUNA SUITS, DIURETICS & DISTILLED WATER

Saunas and Plastic Suits

Let me be clear, if you are wrapping yourself in a plastic suit and locking yourself in an oven, you've already messed up your weight cut. A weight cut performed properly needs nothing more than a pair of bathing trunks and a few friends to have a laugh with. All too often, elite athlete and rank amateur cut weight in the exact same manner through calorie deprivation, dehydration, and exhaustive energy expenditure in extremely hot rooms while dressed like Eskimos. None of this is healthy. And all of this will most certainly reduce your ability to perform.

Distilled Water

Distilled water has been boiled, the vapor captured and restored again to liquid form, devoid of any beneficial elements. Distilled water is very harsh when consumed by humans, especially in cases for prolonged periods of time while at a nutrient deficit. The last thing I want my athletes drinking is distilled water. It will actually force your body to lose more of the vital electrolytes necessary to keep you healthy. Most athletes use distilled water as a means to lose weight and though this may work marginally, its negative effects vastly outweigh the few ounces it may gain you.

Diuretics

Diuretics in most effective forms are illegal in sanctioned competition. Any sort of chemical, prescription, or over-the-counter item must be cleared by all athletic commissions. It is my belief that diuretics cause more damage to the athlete due to the product's aggressive nature and though they do work, it seems very difficult for the athlete to rehydrate effectively and maintain their prior level of health.

This meal plan contains Earth-grown nutrients that have naturally occurring diuretic properties, which allow the body to relieve itself naturally. We always work with the body for maximum benefit.

Natural Diuretics
dandelion
green tea
coffee

KENNY "HULK" PERALTA

Starting weight: 220 lbs. • Ending weight: 145 lbs.

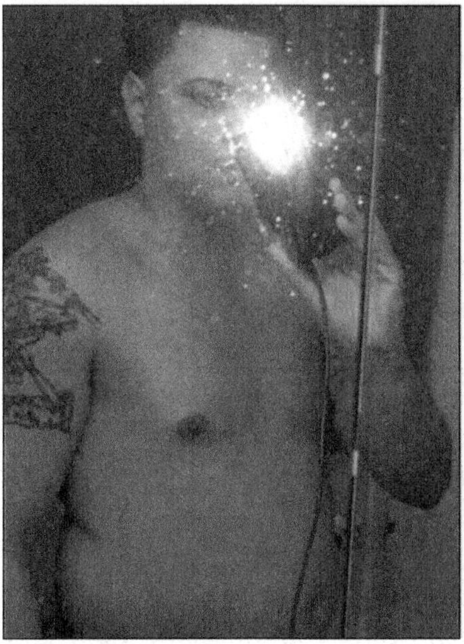
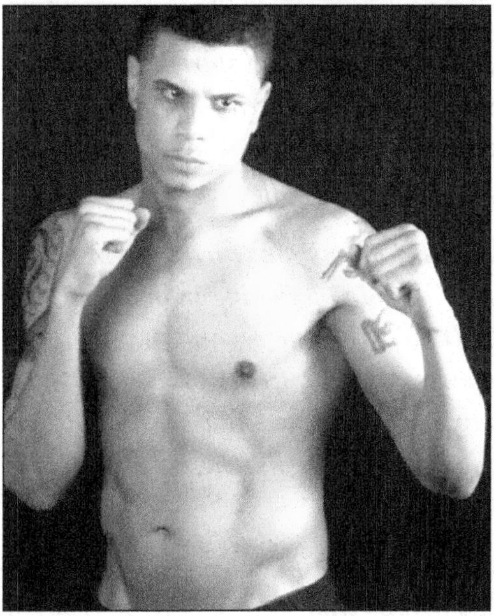

Kenny "Hulk" Peralta before The Dolce Diet at 220 lbs. and after at 145 lbs.

Mike Dolce and Living Lean changed my life. September 2012 I had shoulder surgery to repair a torn labrum. After that happened I could not train and fell into a disgusting binge eating phase where I went from 175 lbs. all the way up to 220. Being only 5'9", I felt disgusted with myself.

March 2013, on my son's first birthday, I couldn't find anything to wear for professional pictures that I felt comfortable in. I tried to hide my weight behind baggy clothes. It took me seeing the pictures and seeing how disgusting I looked to finally say, "That's it. I'm making a change for myself, my health and to have longevity for my son."

Being a fan of MMA I knew about Mike Dolce's success with the top athletes in the world, and not only helping them step on the scale in the best shape, but helping them live better, cleaner lives. I bought Living Lean and Living Lean Cookbook and started my journey. Mind you I never cooked before, so I wasn't an experienced cook of any sort. But I followed the principles and read the simple instructions for the recipes and changed my life, and the weight just began to fly off.

I started on my son's birthday (3/4/13) weighing in at 217 lbs. to one month later (4/4/13) weighing in at 195 lbs. Another month later, (5/4/13) I weighed 180 lbs. Everyone began to notice and I became The Dolce Diet's biggest endorser in Connecticut. Wearing the (Dolce Diet) bag, and with my weight loss, everyone asked how was it possible. I would spread the word as if it was my bible. Before I knew it I had everyone I knew purchasing the books and Living Lean!

It wasn't a diet but a life changer. Changed my life so much that I went for my dreams and took my first MMA fight that summer and weighed in at 155 lbs. It's crazy that I was hitting 220 lbs. 5 months earlier and now I was stepping on the scale at 155 lbs. for my first amateur MMA fight.

But that was just the beginning. I have been on a tear this year with two back-to-back first-round finishes. I even made my 145 lbs. debut in April. It was the easiest weight cut I've ever had. Using 3 Weeks to Shredded, I actually woke up on weight at 145 lbs. Now I'm getting a title fight in July and going pro next year all thanks to The Dolce Diet. I want to personally say thank you to Mike and Brandy for changing my life and giving me the opportunity to follow my dreams.

Respectfully,
Kenny "Hulk" Peralta

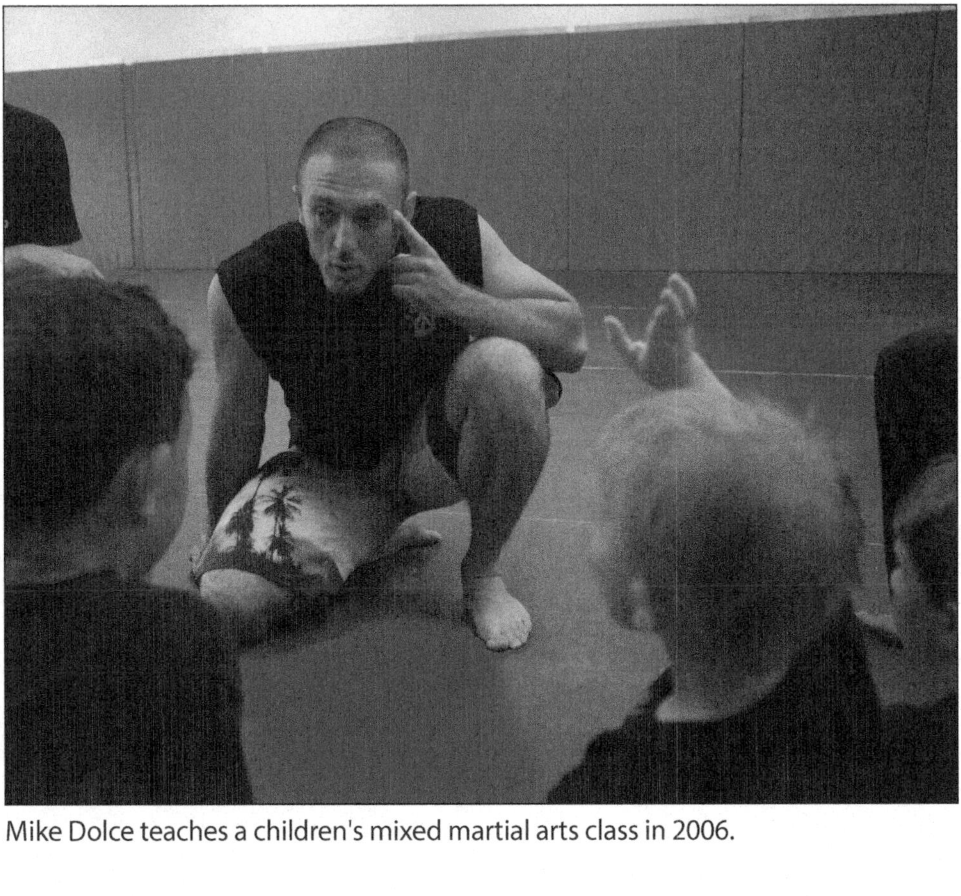

Mike Dolce teaches a children's mixed martial arts class in 2006.

"It takes time to create excellence. If it could be done so quickly, more people would do it." ~John Wooden

TRAVELING DURING THE WEIGHT CUT: HOW TO STAY HEALTHY ON THE ROAD

"The virtue of achievement is victory over oneself. Those who know this can never know defeat." -John Dryden

I created this section to help guide coaches, athletes and those of us dedicated to keeping our bodies healthy and powerfully energetic while away from the comforts and convenience of home.

I'm on the road as much as 250 days a year. That's over 8 months! I have identified the challenges this lifestyle presents and learned to take responsibility for my health by organized planning. I do not allow my hectic schedule to dictate my health.

BE PREPARED

When I pack my luggage, I always bring the following:

- 3 cups of dry oat bran or oatmeal (the equivalent of 12, ¼ cup servings, or the equivalent of 12 meals)
- 3 cups of raisins (can be added to oat bran for a meal or eaten with nuts as a snack; the equivalent of 12, ¼ cup servings)
- 3 cups raw almonds, cashews, peanuts or walnuts
- 3 cups chia seeds
- 3 cups hemp seeds
- 1 stainless steel teaspoon to use anywhere or anytime
- 12 chamomile tea bags (to help me relax before bed)
- 12 green tea bags (to give me a healthy buzz in the early part of the day)
- 1 wide-top, 24 oz. shaker bottle. They make great storage devices for your raisins and nuts while traveling; it allows you to fill up with water at any water fountain or sink; even serves as a handy bowl to make your oat

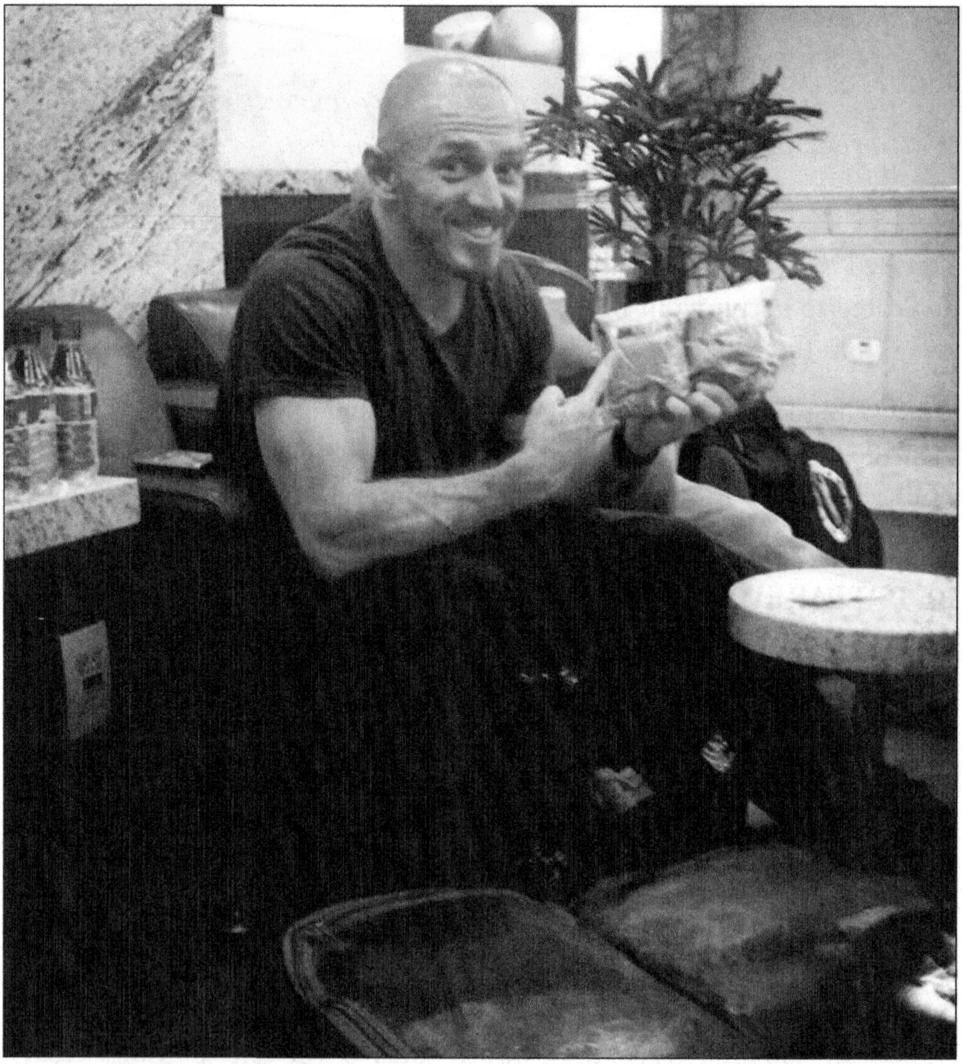

Practicing what he preaches, Coach Mike has all the food he needs packed in his suitcase, which is a good thing during a 16-hour layover in the São Paulo airport.

bran at 2am when you're stranded at some darn airport terminal or when you just walk into your hotel room and are absolutely starving. Again, we are always responsible for our meals.

• I'll throw an apple and an orange in my backpack "just in case."
• I'll bring a handful of ChocoFree Metabolate.
• The above are the essential items to always have with you while traveling. The oat bran will always be ready to eat in any hotel by simply using the coffee maker provided in most every room to heat up some water.

SHOPPING
The next thing I do is find a supermarket or gas station (as a last resort) to grab a few gallons of water for my room, restock my dried fruit (raisins) and raw nuts. I also look for fresh fruits like apples, oranges, bananas, berries and grapes, all of which travel well. You need some sort of essential fat with you to slow down your digestion and give you a sustained energy source while also keeping your cognitive function running smoothly. This is why I bring chia seeds, hemp seeds and raw nuts.

MEALS
Most hotels have a pretty decent menu and you can pretty much always find a nice piece of grilled chicken or fish, some healthy greens like spinach or broccoli, and hearty complex carbs like brown rice and sweet potato. I stay away from white bread, which has a very low nutrient value and can make my insulin spiral out of control. I also avoid margarine and most butters unless it is grass-fed.

When I receive my travel itinerary, I always find out the dining options and room service items before I arrive by looking over the menu online or calling the hotel. Will I be able to use their services, or will I need to make other arrangements? Preparation is most important.

BREAKFAST ON THE ROAD

Breakfast will ALWAYS be oatmeal or oat bran, fresh fruit, lots of water and finished up with a cup of green tea or coffee. This will give your body the necessary fuel to begin your day and switch on your metabolism to begin sustaining your lean muscle and burn any unnecessary body fat.

The common American breakfast relies heavily on bacon, eggs, toast, milk and butter. All of this protein and fat bogs down our digestion and slows down our metabolism, causing a traffic jam in our stomach, and lacks the necessary fuel to prepare our mind and muscles to begin the day.

After a 6-to-8 hour sleep, our body is craving sugar, so that is how we will start. But we will give it very nutrient-dense sugars with additional benefits, like vitamins, minerals, antioxidants, fiber and essential fats, all of which will provide us with the super-fuel we need to hit the day at full power, but with the essential building blocks of life to extend our longevity and repair any free-radical damage that is thrust upon us from daily life.

MID-MEALS

Within 2-to-4 hours, based upon your energy exertion, it will be time to top off your fuel tank with a snack, or what I prefer to call a mid-meal.

A mid-meal may consist of approximately 1/3 the calories and portion size of a standard meal (think breakfast, lunch and dinner) and will typically pair two different energy sources.

I prefer to pair a sugar, like an apple, with an essential fat, like 2 tablespoons of peanut butter / 1 handful of raisins and 1 handful of cashews / or 1 orange and half an avocado.

I look forward to the flavor of my mid-meals and value the mood enhancing benefit it has on me by stabilizing my sinking blood sugar levels.

DINNER

At dinner, it is common in America to consume a piece of protein (steak, chicken, fish) that takes up 2/3 of the plate with the remaining 1/3 being a complex carbohydrate like a potato or rice. Green vegetables are usually crammed in there somewhere as an afterthought.

I prefer half of the plate to be green vegetables (the more alive the better), 1/4 of the plate for protein and 1/4 for complex carbs.

This is much more in line with what our body actually needs and less in line with what television commercials and other mass marketing tells us we should want.

While traveling, stick to the "Lean and Green." Lean proteins are chicken, fish and plant-based foods, and stick with greens like spinach, broccoli, asparagus and Brussels sprouts. Remember your goals, and stay focused.

DANIEL GONZALEZ

Starting weight: 200 lbs. • Ending weight: 155 lbs.

My whole family was overweight, have diabetes and was unhealthy. I was 200 lbs. and I didn't want to fall into illness as my family did, so I decided to buy The Dolce Diet and follow the guidelines. By eating six times a day and never missing breakfast, I lost 45 lbs. and am in great shape.

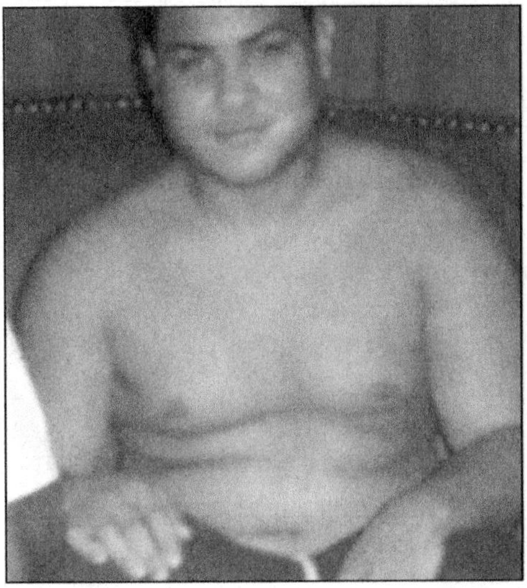

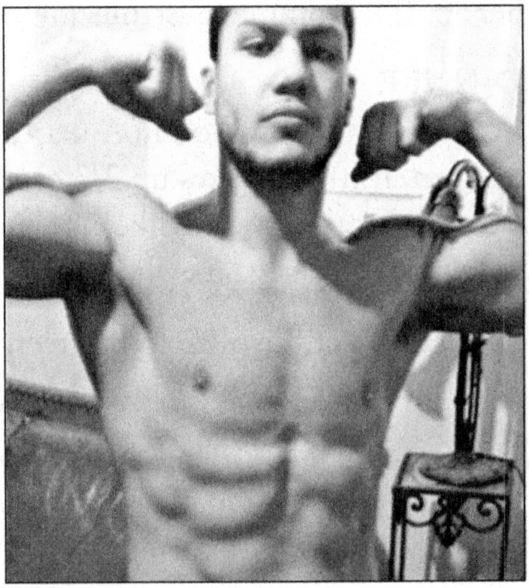

Daniel Gonzalez before The Dolce Diet at 200 lbs. and after at 155 lbs.

"In order to grow we must be open to new ideas…new ways of doing things… new ways of thinking." ~*George Raveling*

TRAINING WHILE CUTTING WEIGHT

This is one of the great misconceptions during fight week. Training itself is a rigorous task all of which should have been completed in the 8 weeks prior to fight week. Fight week itself is dedicated to peaking, to performing the necessary tasks related to the promotion of an organized event. Fight week is also dedicated to weight cutting, which is the main topic of this book. You can train like a world-class athlete with everything perfectly performed for 8 weeks and throw it all away during fight week because you trained too hard and depleted your body to the point that it reached a level of being unrecoverable in the short period of time you have until fight night.

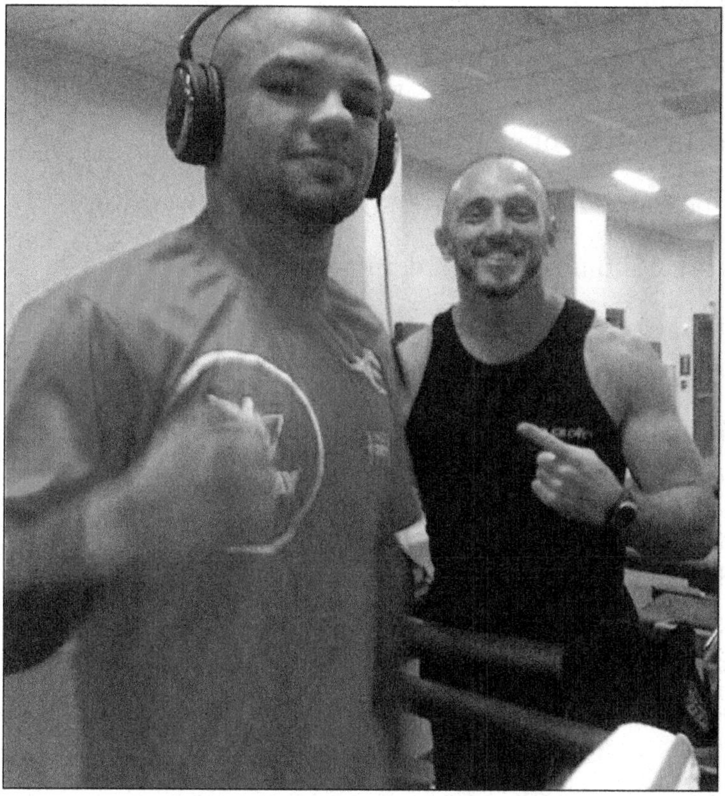

Thiago "Pitbull" Alves completes a light treadmill session during fight week.

I strongly suggest athletes do not train at all during fight week. General activity should be embraced. One of my favorite parts of fight trips is to explore the city with my athlete and their team. These are the types of activities and exercises we perform to maintain a vibrant level of health.

Done are the days of sparring and sprinting and shrimping and striking. Now is the time to relax, recover, repair and reset. We prepare the body to lose weight through healthy methods by eating highly nutritious foods, by maintaining adequate hydration levels, and by balancing our rest with our exertion.

Some athletes for psychological reasons like to go over their game plans during fight week. This is fine, if conducted under direct supervision while adhering to a specific set of guidelines.

- The session must be short. 20-30 minutes max including warm-up.
- The athlete's heart rate should not exceed 140 bpm.
- The athlete should not work at a rate that forces him or her to take a deep breath.
- All activity should be done in a manner that would allow complete conversations to be had.

These points are very important. Many of the old-school or uninformed around the sport don't understand this process. They believe it's best to put on plastic suits and warm-up jackets and hit the pads hard for an hour and grapple for an hour and heck, maybe even spar. Some even do this as a regular part of their weight-cutting routine. Absurd!

The whole point to these sessions is only because the athlete needs psychological reassurance. This is a psychological workout; a cognitive workout. This is not a physical workout. These athletes are multimillion-dollar machines that need to be scientifically calibrated during fight week, not put on the track and run in the red line until something rattles loose!

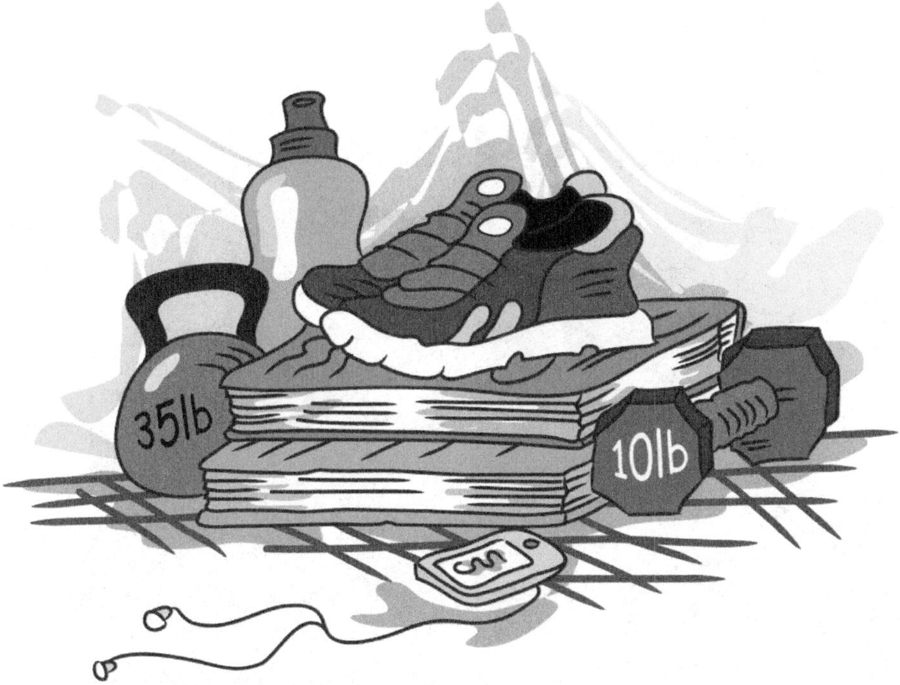

PHILLIP DASILVA

Starting weight: 175 lbs. • Ending weight: 160 lbs.

I am an amateur Muay Thai competitor and have been competing for the last 4 years. I always struggled with getting my weight down for competitions. Being only 5'6", my original goal was to compete at 160 lbs. I had early success, winning my fights early on. But my diet consisted of only brown rice, chicken, broccoli and egg whites.

Most days, I was just so sick of the food that I would cheat very often and feel terrible. I struggled mentally with my diet until I came across Mike Dolce. Then my life and mood changed significantly. My goal to compete at 147 lbs. would never have been possible without 3 Weeks to Shredded! My next goal is 140 lbs.! BOOM!

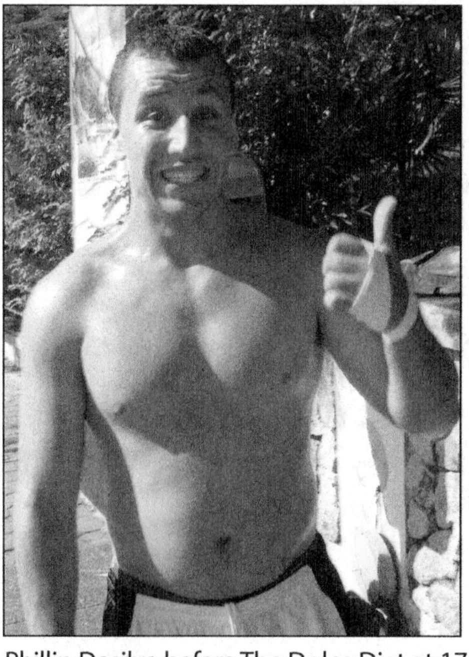

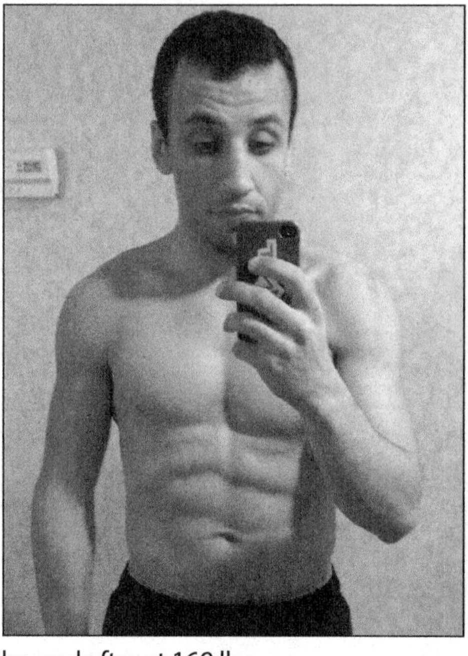

Phillip Dasilva before The Dolce Diet at 175 lbs. and after at 160 lbs.

"A coach must never forget that he is a leader and not merely a person with authority." ~John Wooden

EXPECTATIONS: THE COACH / ATHLETE RELATIONSHIP

We have to understand that the coach / athlete relationship is the most important bond during fight week. The closer we get to performance the less external influences we should allow. The coach's main responsibility is ensuring the athlete has every single thing he needs to perform at his peak potential and in a healthy manner.

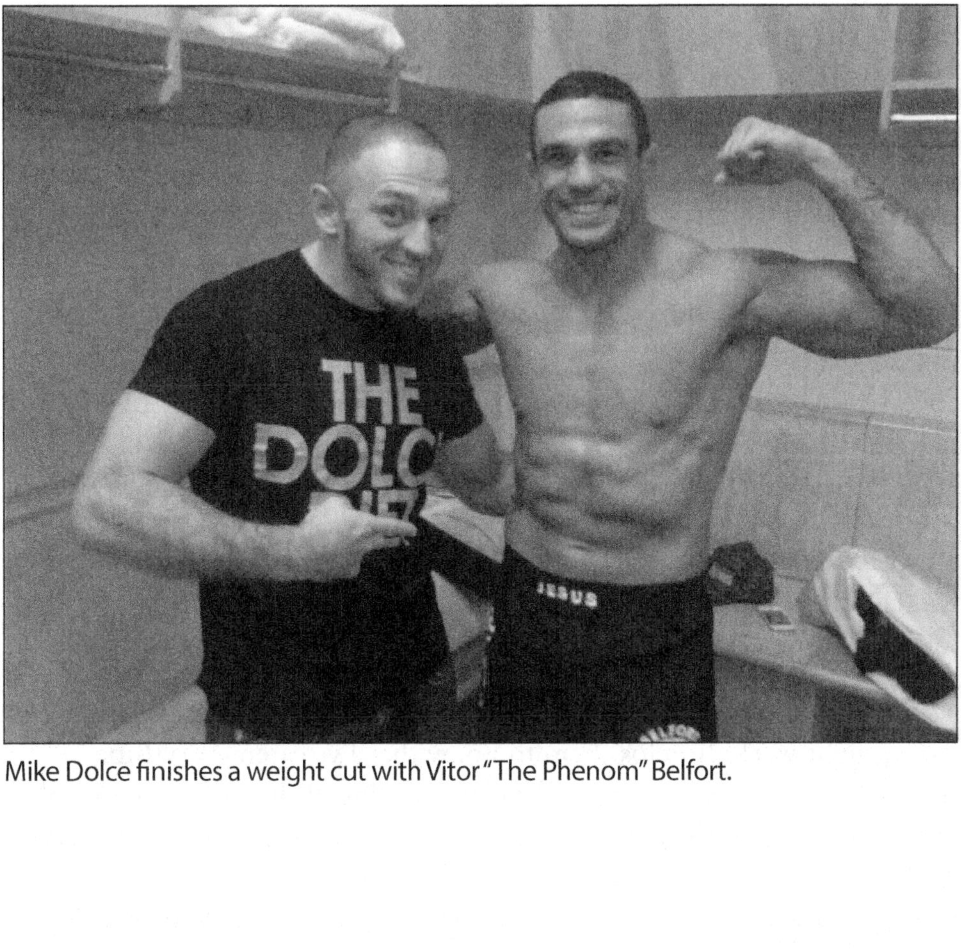

Mike Dolce finishes a weight cut with Vitor "The Phenom" Belfort.

All too often I see athletes struggling during fight week, suffering through rigorous training sessions on limited calories and drinking little-to-no water. Meanwhile the coaches are carrying lattes and colas, eating cheeseburgers and even pizzas. Oftentimes they are making fun of the athlete to "toughen up" or asking "doesn't this smell good?" and "Don't worry! You can have this on Saturday."

What benefit does that give the athlete? Many athletes are accustomed to this, and it doesn't offend them nearly as much as it offends me. They've grown accustomed to being abused. In spite of this, they are able to perform at adequate levels, but certainly not at their peak potential. When I work with an athlete, I do everything my athlete does and more.

If he wakes up at 6am, I wake up at 5am to ensure the day is prepared. This allows the athlete the ability to focus 100 percent on the task at hand. What my athlete eats, I eat. And one step further, I hand-prepare everything. I do all the grocery shopping. I don't go to the hotel cafe in the lobby like many of the other teams. I'll fly into town a day or two before the athlete to locally source all the ingredients necessary. These ingredients could be spinach, cherries or international battery adapters and cooking skillets. Most of the other coaches don't even bring an apple for the 18-hour flight. I say all this because I've seen it happen firsthand.

Typically, I lose lb. for lb. the same amount of weight as my athlete during fight week. It helps them to know that I've eaten everything they've eaten and not one morsel more. I've sipped the same amount of water; I've gone to the press conference, and I've hopped on the airplanes. And I've sweat drip for drip the same amount they have. So as we roll deeper into fight week, and closer to the scale, the athlete knows he isn't alone. Climbing into a cage to fight another man is a very lonely prospect. For me, I try to offer every possible advantage to my athlete.

And if losing 20 lbs. in 4 days alongside them offers .001 percent advantage, I'm more than happy to do it. That's well worth the trade-off for me.

Recently at an event in Canada, I was in the hot tub with one of my athletes on Wednesday relaxing and breaking a good sweat. We were both fully fed and hydrated sipping away on our gallon jugs of purified water mixed with chia seeds and fresh-squeezed lime, and another athlete competing on the same card was in the tub looking terrible. He was all alone, and had only 6 more lbs. to lose to make the lightweight limit. My athlete was 16 lbs. above the lightweight limit, but looked amazing. He was telling jokes and acting out previous fights as if he hadn't a care in the world. We stayed in the hot tub an hour longer to not leave this other kid all alone, who was struggling.

About halfway into the soak, this kid's coaches come walking into the spa. They say hello, ask their guy how he's doing and then crack some jokes about how he looks like a skeleton. One of the coaches, a little more fit and a little quieter than the rest, walks around the massive hot tub to where I was immersed and says, "Why do you do this?" I looked at him quizzically and asked, "What do you mean?" He said, "Why do you keep yourself in such good shape and cut weight with the athletes the way you do? I've seen you before with different athletes doing this."
I looked at him and said, "Why wouldn't I?"

My whole job is to help this kid win. I'm 100 percent dedicated to my athletes, my clients, my students, my craft, my integrity. It breaks my heart when I see these guys and girls suffering all alone packed in plastic bags, zip-tied in woolen cotton and set to bake in these wooden ovens while their apathetic coaches stand outside the door and make jokes.

Athletes, hear me now: YOU are the boss. The Bill Gates, the Lorenzo Fertitta of your company. Your coaches are part of your executive staff. They are hired for a very specific and elite skill set, but they answer to YOU! Especially during fight week, which is the whole point of the last 3 months of training. If your coaches do not conduct themselves 100 percent as professionals, dedicated to your success and well-being, they should be put on notice immediately.

With that said and with this book, I cannot foresee any athlete, any coach, any team, acting in a manner counterproductive to your joint successes. That is why I'm giving you this information, to see you all perform at your best possible levels, while maintaining an extreme state of health. I'm asking you to all please recognize that this is the primary goal.

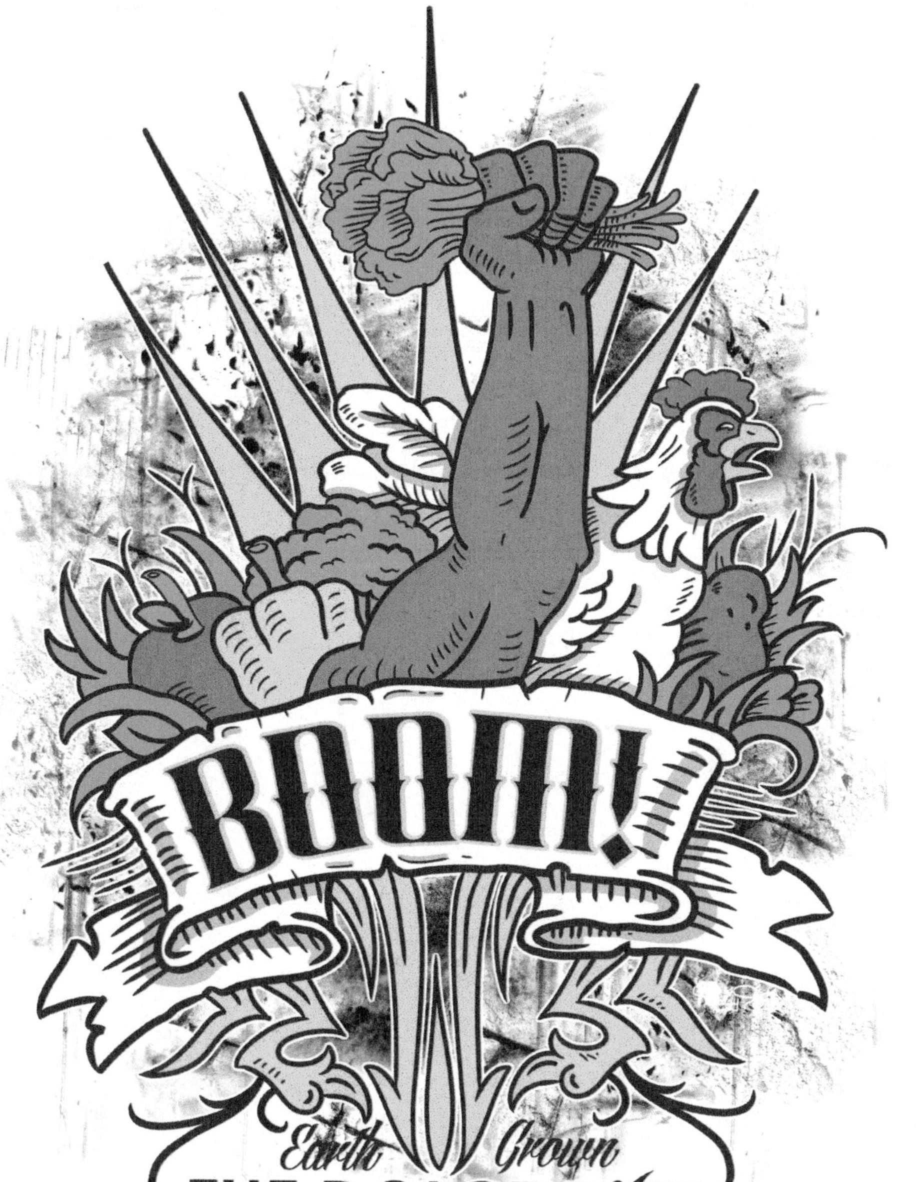
BOOM!
Earth Grown
THE DOLCE DIET

Appendix

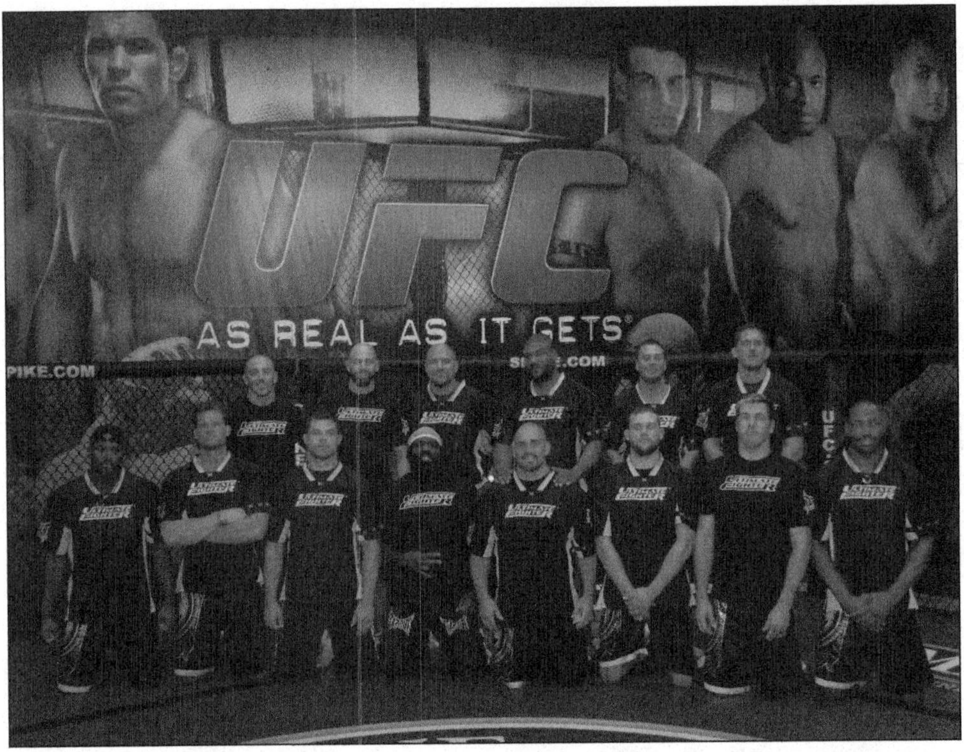

Mike Dolce and the Season 10 team of "The Ultimate Fighter," - the most watched season of the series.

GROCERY LIST:
THE ORIGINAL 3 WEEKS TO SHREDDED

Egg whites
Turkey bacon
Chicken breast
Salmon

Spinach
Tomato
Onion
Dill pickle

Apple
Pear
Dried cranberries
Mixed berries
Applesauce

Oatmeal

Purified water
Green Tea
Tropicana Orange Juice with Calcium and Vitamin D Added
Flax Oil
Grapeseed oil
Extra Virgin Olive Oil
Smart Balance Buttery Spread with Flax Added
Whey protein

GROCERY LIST:
THE NEW 3 WEEKS TO SHREDDED

Always purchase organic, grass-fed products when available.

Eggs
Blue cheese crumbles
Black beans
Turkey bacon
Chicken breast
Steak
Salmon

Spinach
Kale
Tomato
Red onion
Red pepper
Green pepper
Asparagus
Garlic cloves

Apples
Oranges
Pears
Raisins
Blueberries
Mixed berries (fresh seasonal fruit)
Applesauce
Avocado

Oat bran
Ezekiel bread

Chia seeds
Hemp seeds
Amaranth
Almonds
Almond butter (both salted & unsalted)

Purified water
Green tea
Coffee
Coconut water

Avocado oil
Coconut oil
Extra virgin olive oil
Balsamic vinegar
Cinnamon
Honey
Pink Himalayan sea salt

Vitamin C
Dandelion root
Uva ursi
Post workout protein (see TheDolceDiet.com for Dolce Diet Approved proteins.)
ChocoFree Metabolate (onnit.com/dolce)

MORE RESOURCES

TWITTER
Follow Mike Dolce on Twitter **@TheDolceDiet** and read his "favorited tweets" for inspirational testimonials!

FACEBOOK
Check out The Dolce Diet fan page at **Facebook.com/TheDolceDiet**

YOUTUBE
For videos detailing exercises, recipes and so much more, visit The Dolce Diet YouTube channel at **YouTube.com/dolcediet**

THE DOLCE DIET SOCIAL NETWORK
It's FREE! Design your own profile page at **MYDolceDiet.com** and talk with Mike during his frequent LIVE CHATS, as well as with others living healthy, vibrant lifestyles just like you!

THE DOLCE DIET OFFICIAL WEBSITE
Get the latest news about Mike, his athletes, health tips and more at **TheDolceDiet.com**

THE MIKE DOLCE SHOW
Mike answers your questions and chats with featured guests weekly! Listen at **TheMikeDolceShow.com**, on iTunes or Stitcher, or by downloading our free Android and Apple iOS apps!

THE DOLCE DIET SHOP
Clothing, books, bags and more! Visit **DolceDietShop.com** today.

BOOKS BY MIKE DOLCE

#1 Bestseller The Dolce Diet: LIVING LEAN
#1 Bestseller The Dolce Diet: LIVING LEAN COOKBOOK
#1 Bestseller The Dolce Diet: COLLEGE DIET GUIDE
Available in paperback & ebook at **amazon.com** worldwide and in ebook at iTunes (iBooks.)

Exercise DVDs by Mike Dolce
UFC FIT - 12-week training program with nutrition and lifestyle manual.
Available at **UFCFIT.com**

For more information about Mike Dolce & The Dolce Diet visit **TheDolceDiet.com**

CPSIA information can be obtained
at www.ICGtesting.com
Printed in the USA
FSOW03n2254090417
32837FS

9 780984 963188